CONCISE GUIDE TO

Treatment of Alcoholism and Addictions

Second Edition

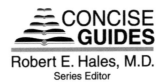

CONCISE GUIDES

Robert E. Hales, M.D.

Series Editor

CONCISE GUIDE TO
Treatment of Alcoholism and Addictions

Second Edition

Avram H. Mack, M.D.
Resident Physician, The Brigham and Women's Hospital
Clinical Fellow, Harvard Medical School
Boston, Massachusetts

John E. Franklin Jr., M.D., M.Sc.
Associate Professor of Psychiatry and
Director, Addiction Psychiatry,
Northwestern University School of Medicine
Chicago, Illinois

Richard J. Frances, M.D.
President and Medical Director,
Silver Hill Hospital, New Canaan, Connecticut
Clinical Professor of Psychiatry, New York University
Adjunct Professor of Psychiatry,
University of Medicine and Dentistry of New Jersey
Newark, New Jersey

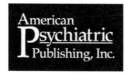

American Psychiatric Publishing, Inc.

Washington, DC
London, England

Copyright © 2001 American Psychiatric Publishing, Inc.
ALL RIGHTS RESERVED

Manufactured in the United States of America on acid-free paper
08 07 06 05   5 4 3 2
Second Edition

American Psychiatric Publishing, Inc.
1000 Wilson Boulevard
Arlington, VA 22209-3901
www.appi.org

Library of Congress Cataloging-in-Publication Data
Mack, Avram H.
   Concise guide to treatment of alcoholism and addictions / Avram H. Mack, John E.
Franklin, Jr., Richard J. Frances.—2nd ed.
      p. ; cm.
   Rev. ed. of: Concise guide to treatment of alcoholism and addictions / Richard J. Frances,
John E. Franklin, Jr.
   Includes bibliographical references and index.
   ISBN 0-88048-803-4 (alk. paper)
      1. Substance abuse—Treatment—Handbooks, manuals, etc. 2. Alcoholism—Treatment—
Handbooks, manuals, etc. I. Franklin, John E., 1954– II. Frances, Richard J. III. Frances,
Richard J. Concise guide to treatment of alcoholism and addictions. IV. Title.
      [DNLM: 1. Alcoholism—therapy—Handbooks. 2. Substance-Related Disorders—therapy—
Handbooks. WM 34 M153c 2001]
   RC564.F73 2001
   616.86′06—dc21

                                                                                    00-067644

British Library Cataloguing in Publication Data
A CIP record is available from the British Library.

To our mothers:
Marsha Mack Frances, Arlena T. Franklin, and Julia Frances,
and to all mothers who are in support of addiction treatment

CONTENTS

List of Tables

INTRODUCTION

to the Concise Guides Series

The Concise Guides Series from American Psychiatric Publishing, Inc., provides, in an accessible format, practical information for psychiatrists, psychiatry residents, and medical students working in a variety of treatment settings, such as inpatient psychiatry units, outpatient clinics, consultation-liaison services, and private office settings. The Concise Guides are meant to complement the more detailed information that is found in lengthier psychiatry texts.

The Concise Guides address topics of special concern to psychiatrists in clinical practice. The books in this series contain a detailed table of contents, along with an index, tables, figures, and other charts for easy access. The books are designed to fit into a lab coat pocket or jacket pocket, which makes them a convenient source of information. References have been limited to those most relevant to the material presented.

Robert E. Hales, M.D., M.B.A.
Series Editor, Concise Guides

PREFACE

In the United States, substance use disorders (SUDs) present a tremendous medical and social challenge: 13.8% of all Americans will have an alcohol-related SUD in their life, an estimated 14.8 million Americans were current users of illicit drugs in 1999, and including the related aspects of crime, absenteeism, and treatment, the monetary cost to the nation is estimated to be greater than $275 billion annually. Those in every category of health care—physicians, nurses, psychologists, social workers, alcohol and drug counselors, and rehabilitation therapists, as well as students in all of these areas—are constantly faced with treatment choices and options that are critical to the care of patients with SUDs.

This handbook is designed to be a concise guide containing useful tools for the choices and options of treatment employed by these professionals. Although primarily written with the clinician in mind, many allied helping professions such as the clergy, educators, lawyers, police officers, and corrections personnel will find the book useful. Education about addictions has been increasing recently for health professionals. Yet, considering the magnitude of the problem, this area remains underrepresented in the core of medical student and resident curriculums, and both generalist and specialist training is needed for nurses, social workers, and psychologists. Addiction counselors need more psychiatric training to better deal with comorbidity.

This extensively revised second edition is a concise overview of addiction treatment issues, is relevant to the clinician in the trenches, and is a distillation of our clinical experience as well as our review of the literature. This second edition is improved by the suggestions of the readers of the first edition. During a 24-year period at The New York Hospital, New Jersey Medical School, Hackensack Hospital, and Silver Hill Hospital, Richard Frances, M.D., has had the opportunity to follow the treatment course and progress of 5,000 inpatients with substance disorders and to supervise approximately 1,000 psychiatric residents, both individually and in their teams. As founding president of the American Academy of Addiction Psychiatry and as chair of the American Psychiatric Association Council on the Addictions, he has been a leader in the field. At Cornell, the New Jersey Medical School, and Northwestern Medical Center, John Franklin, M.D., has worked extensively with inpatient, outpatient, and consultation service treatment planning for this population and has developed a special interest in patients requiring organ transplant. A resident at the Harvard-Longwood Program, Avram H. Mack, M.D., provides the perspective of a trainee who is also a Trustee of the American Psychiatric Association.

The limitations of a handbook format, in terms of summarizing and highlighting the important issues, led us to focus on what we feel is the most important clinically relevant material, at the risk of omitting extensive presentations of research data and reviews of literature. We are grateful to Robert Hales, M.D., Carol Nadelson, M.D., and Ron McMillen for their suggestions regarding the book; to our colleagues, staff, teachers, and students at the New York Hospital–Cornell Medical Center, the New Jersey Medical School, New York University Medical School, Silver Hill Hospital, Northwestern University Medical Center, the Brigham and Women's Hospital, the Massachusetts Mental Health Center, the Beth Israel Deaconess Medical Center, and Harvard Medical School; and to our patients who have worked with us in understanding treatment problems. In addition, George Vaillant, M.D., John Renner, M.D., Joseph Scavetta, M.D., Allen Frances, M.D., Jonathan Borus, M.D., William E. Greenberg, M.D., and Jeremy R. Mack, M.D., have provided invaluable support and guidance. We also thank Elizabeth Lopato for her patience, assistance, and editorial comments in preparing the manuscript for the second edition. Finally, without encouragement from Day, Arline, and Marsha the work would not have been possible.

Avram H. Mack, M.D.
John E. Franklin Jr., M.D., M.Sc.
Richard J. Frances, M.D.

INTRODUCTION

This guide to the treatment of substance use disorders (SUDs) disseminates the implications of new research on addiction treatment and a variety of approaches that have been useful to clinicians. Patients, their families, and clinicians face confusing choices about treatment combinations that should be tailored to the individual. Answers about optimal treatment combinations await valid and well-constructed outcome research; the current literature on SUD treatment outcome is relatively sparse, nonspecific, and of limited usefulness to the clinician. The clinician's choices are enhanced by a careful history, by mental status and physical examinations, by diagnostic formulation, and by confirmatory evidence from laboratory tests and third-party sources. The American Psychiatric Association (APA) practice guidelines on SUDs and the American Society of Addiction Medicine (ASAM) placement criteria provide general guides to this uncharted territory (1, 2) as does the recent National Institute on Drug Abuse guide (3). In addition, this extensively updated and revised second edition of this *Concise Guide* was created for the clinician seeking practical, direct advice about common problems in the field. This chapter outlines some of the most essential points in this increasingly complex field. A note at the outset: *Substance use disorders,* which are defined in DSM-IV-TR (4) and described in Chapter 4 of this book, is a term that employs the word *use. Use* is not interchangeable with *abuse* or *dependence* and a definitive diagnosis is always important.

Treatment of SUDs can be extremely difficult. Helping the patient to recognize a problem and to accept help are the two most important steps in treatment, recognized both by self-help groups and by research concerning motivational interviewing and stages of awareness (5). These two steps are frequently difficult because of the nature of addictive disorders, which leads to denial, lying, and organicity (central nervous system pathology). Both patient and therapist may struggle with the stigma of substance disorders and with accepting that the patient has an illness. Most patients will wish to achieve controlled use and will have difficulty accepting the therapist's standard of abstinence as the goal for treatment. Patients frequently feel hopeless about ever achieving sustained abstinence and need to be encouraged that the goal is attainable. Seeing others who are recovering and personal experience of increasing periods of abstinence help improve hope. Harm avoidance approaches such as needle exchange, relapse prevention, and continuance of pharmacological and psychotherapeutic modalities for patients with comorbidity can be combined with a long-range goal of abstinence. Unfortunately, the term *harm avoidance* is also used sometimes as part of the justification for legalization of illicit substances, a position we oppose. Legalization would increase availability and lower the costs of drugs, and it would increase the number of complications and comorbidity of SUDs. Prevention and treatment should be made more widely available to reduce use, and drug courts should be alternatives to the traditional justice system. More treatment should be available to prisoners as well. Drug substitution (e.g., methadone or buprenorphine maintenance) and the use of other indicated medications may be met with resistance that will often need to be worked through.

■ GENERAL TENETS OF THE TREATMENT OF SUDS

1. *Case heterogeneity*. Patients are individuals and vary in terms of the substance(s) they use and their pattern of use, severity of abuse or dependence, functional impairment, secondary medical conditions, psychiatric comorbidity, personal strengths and vulnerabilities, and social and environmental context. Thus no one treatment works for all individuals.

2. *Phases of treatment.* Active treatment progresses: results do not happen all at once. Begin with comprehensive assessment and move to treatment of intoxication or withdrawal, development of a treatment plan, and enactment of the plan. The amount of time in treatment is a critical prognostic factor.

3. *Comprehensiveness.* Assessment and treatment must take into account all aspects of the individual's life and illness. Collateral sources of information are extremely important in assessment. Coexisting psychiatric and medical conditions should be treated concurrently in an integrated manner. Treatment programs should assess for HIV, hepatitis, tuberculosis, and other infectious diseases and should provide education to help patients to reduce their risk of contracting communicable diseases.

4. *Treatment plans.* Goals of treatment should include the reduction of substance use, the achievement of abstinence, the infrequency of relapse, and rehabilitation and recovery. Treatment status must be continually reviewed, reassessed, and updated.

5. *View of relapse.* Relapses occur; all treatment plans must include assessment of relapses. They do not always imply treatment failure. Treatment must continue, but the need for increased surveillance must be addressed. Abstinence may sometimes seem an impossible goal (e.g., in the elderly), but reductions in morbidity and mortality follow any reduction in substance use, which makes the effort worthwhile (6).

■ THE THERAPEUTIC ALLIANCE

The therapeutic alliance may be one of the clinician's most important tools. Having frequently grown up in families with SUDs, patients with substance use problems are, not surprisingly, likely to have typical transference resistances to treatment and are likely to evoke countertransference reactions in the therapist that may either facilitate or negate treatment, depending on how the reactions are handled (7). Therapists who are well informed and well trained and who understand and are in touch with their own

---

TABLE 1–1.   **Attributes and attitudes helpful in working with patients with substance use disorders**

---

1. Respect the provision of a caring and compassionate relationship.
2. The therapist should be an informed optimist.
3. The therapist needs the capacity to tolerate his or her own anxiety, pain, frustration, and depression.
4. Have flexibility and open-mindedness.
5. Possess good knowledge of general psychiatry, resourcefulness, and creativity.
6. Have intellectual curiosity.
7. The best therapists possess wisdom.
8. Have persistence and patience.
9. Cultivate the capacity to listen and to watch both what is and what is not said and to act accordingly.
10. Honesty and integrity are important in the therapist and in the treatment team.

---

feelings are more helpful to patients and are less likely to experience ''burnout'' (8). We can think of 10 attributes and attitudes that are helpful in working with patients with SUDs. These are summarized in Table 1–1.

1. The most crucial nonspecific variable is an attitude of respect for the provision of a caring and compassionate relationship. Often underestimated, a concern for patients and a willingness to form an active therapeutic alliance (with some degree of therapeutic zeal but without overidentification) are crucial when working with patients who have SUDs. An empathic capacity to feel the patient's experience and yet to maintain objectivity is crucial. Following a tradition in psychotherapy (which goes back to Ferenczi and Alexander) of activity and of creating an environment in which a patient can achieve comfort and growth is desirable. This approach includes an ability to confront with concern as well as to provide emotional support appropriately, which of course does not mean playing a real sexual or parental role or taking on a contrived position that is not genuinely felt by the therapist. It is important that the therapist not abuse the power that the patient invests in him or her, but rather exercise it with decency and compassion.

2. The therapist should be an informed optimist. It has been said that the difference between an optimist and a pessimist is that the pessimist is better informed. However, therapeutic nihilism or over-identification with a patient's helplessness, low self-esteem, and hopelessness often contributes to poor treatment results. An informed optimism based on knowledge of the course and treatment of addictions and on the experience of working with patients who have done well is a tremendous asset to any therapist. Acceptance of the limits of treatment and of the chronic nature of SUDs, however, is equally important.

3. The therapist's capacity to tolerate anxiety, pain, frustration, and depression is essential and may aid in the patient being able to identify with these feelings without resorting to substance use. When therapists are unaware of their own weaknesses and sensitive areas, they may find themselves colluding with the patient in the avoidance of painful areas. Therapists who know themselves and can tolerate depression are also able to work with patients with more difficult challenges.

4. Flexibility and open-mindedness are desirable therapist traits. Simple answers to complicated problems applied uniformly without taking into account special circumstances are often wrong. When therapists and treatment programs hold dogmatic positions, the result is often blind spots, the facilitation of splitting, and the re-creation of an atmosphere of conflict already familiar in patients' lives. Flexibility can involve bringing together several modalities of treatment, the sequential use of clinical trials of different modalities, and willingness to seek out consultation and supervision in difficult cases. The setting of strict limits and providing consistency of approach can be implemented along with the kind of flexibility discussed here.

5. In addition to good knowledge of general psychiatry, resourcefulness, creativity, and knowledge about a number of modalities of treatment are extremely helpful.

6. Intellectual curiosity is vital to the therapist's growth. It is essential that the therapist keep up with the clinical and research literature. The therapist should have an active interest and curiosity in learning more about the needs of each patient.

7. The best therapists possess wisdom. This may grow with the therapist's work and life experience and is enhanced by humility and a sense of humor. Many fine therapists use metaphors in ways that capture an image of immense usefulness to the patient. The eminent behavioral psychologist Howard Hunt once told a patient, who was acting out and abusing multiple substances, that he was behaving like a loose cannon on the deck of a rolling wooden ship in a storm. Another time he compared a patient with self-defeating behaviors and alcoholism to a child who was always reaching for ice cream cones only to have them melt before they reached his lips. Perhaps wisdom is best stated in the serenity prayer, which seeks ''serenity to accept the things I cannot change, courage to change the things I can, and wisdom to know the difference.''

8. Persistence and patience are qualities that are as valuable to clinicians as they are to researchers. Like a fisherman chasing a marlin, the therapist must be able to wait, to work hard, and to be prepared for either little or late ultimate gratification.

9. The capacity to listen and to watch both what is and what is not said and to act accordingly is very important. This includes sharing with the patient what has been heard. ''You listen but you don't hear,'' ''you don't listen,'' ''you aren't seeing what I am really like,'' may or may not be said to the therapist. The statements may be true, or they may represent the way the patient felt about parents or other figures in the patient's life. Because of denial, signs and symptoms of problems need to be closely watched. In the SUD field, perhaps because of the emphasis on psychoeducation and counseling, the basic skills of listening always need to be emphasized.

10. Honesty and integrity in the therapist and in the treatment team are crucial. Extremely sensitive to deception and frequently mistrustful, the patient will need to have an ongoing consistent experience with a therapist worthy of trust. In working with patients with SUDs who have experienced a regression or erosion of their value systems, examination of values almost inevitably becomes part of treatment. The therapist's integrity becomes an important asset in this exploration. Common and sometimes sub-

TABLE 1–2. **Abuses in the treatment of substance use disorders**

1. Preferential treatment influenced by VIP pressures, resulting in mistakes and splitting in the team
2. Distortions of diagnosis (e.g., underdiagnosis of alcoholism because of fears or pressure)
3. Premature discharge to save money
4. Ordering of excessive laboratory tests or diagnostic measures and overcharging for services
5. Excessively punitive or critical approaches, with constant threats of discharge in patients who are resistant to treatment
6. Breaches of confidentiality, leading to major problems in trust

tle forms of corruption of the treatment can occur and must be carefully avoided. The team approach frequently can lead to an open and honest discussion, which may help individuals face their own countertransference issues and may strengthen the total treatment approach.

■ POTENTIAL ABUSES IN THE TREATMENT OF SUDS

Table 1–2 includes examples of more or less subtle forms of corruption that individual therapists and treatment programs must attempt to avoid and to manage if they occur.

■ REFERENCES

1. Work Group on Substance Use Disorders: Practice guideline for the treatment of patients with substance use disorders: alcohol, cocaine, opioids. Am J Psychiatry 152:1a–59a, 1995
2. American Society of Addiction Medicine: Patient Placement Criteria for the Treatment of Substance-Related Disorders, 2nd Edition. Chevy Chase, MD, American Society of Addiction Medicine, 1996

3. National Institute on Drug Abuse: Principles of Drug Addiction Treatment: A Research-Based Guide (NIDA Publication 99-4180). Rockville, MD, National Institute on Drug Abuse, 1999

4. American Psychiatric Association: Diagnostic and Statistical Manual of Mental Disorders, 4th Edition, Text Revision. Washington, DC, American Psychiatric Association, 2000

5. Prochaska JO, DiClemente CC, Norcross JC: In search of how people change: applications to addictive behavior. Am Psychol 47:1102–1114, 1992

6. Marlatt GA, Gordon JR: Relapse Prevention: Maintenance Strategies in the Treatment of Addictive Behaviors. New York, Guilford Press, 1985

7. Group for the Advancement of Psychiatry: Addiction Treatment: Avoiding Pitfalls—A Case Approach (GAP Report 142). Washington, DC, American Psychiatric Press, 1998

8. Frances RJ, Alexopoulos GS: Patient management and education: getting the alcoholic into treatment. Physician and Patient 1:9–14, 1982

MAGNITUDE OF THE PROBLEM

■ GENERAL EPIDEMIOLOGY

Substance use disorders (SUDs) are likely the most prevalent of all types of medical and mental disorders, and they cost society greatly. This chapter focuses on the epidemiology of SUDs. There are a number of studies from which we have gathered most of our data: the Drug Abuse Warning Network (DAWN) (1), which provides ongoing surveillance data, the Monitoring the Future study (2), an ongoing study of substance abuse among American high school and college students and young adults, the National Household Survey (NHS) (3), the Epidemiologic Catchment Area (ECA) study (4), and the National Comorbidity Survey (NCS) (5). Despite a massive effort at interdiction, prevention, and treatment, by almost all measures, substance abuse is not waning in the United States (although use among youth ages 12–17 has decreased since 1997).

■ FACTS OF GENERAL MAGNITUDE

- In 1999, 14.8 million Americans were current users of illicit drugs, up from 13.6 million in 1998 (3).
- In 1999 an estimated 3.6 million Americans met diagnostic criteria for dependence on illicit drugs, and 1.1 million were youths ages 12–17 (3).
- Drug abuse deaths reported to DAWN increased from 9,565 to 10,091 between 1997 and 1998 (1).

- Use varies by age to a great degree, and the rates of use are changing. Current use by youths ages 12–17 is declining: 11.4% of youths ages 12–17 in 1997, 9.9% in 1998, and 9.0% in 1999. The rate was highest (16.3%) in 1979, declined to 5.3% in 1992, and has fluctuated since. Unfortunately, at the same time, use by young adults (ages 18–25) increased from 14.7% in 1997 to 18.8% in 1999 (3).
- The prevalence of youth marijuana use did not change significantly between 1997 and 1998, when it was 9.4% and 8.3%, respectively. Youth use peaked in 1979 at 14.2% and declined to 3.4% in 1992 but grew to 8.2% between 1992 and 1995 and has fluctuated since then (7.1% in 1996 and 9.4% in 1997) (3).
- An estimated 1.5 million (0.7%) Americans ages 12 and older were current users of cocaine in 1999. Cocaine use reached a peak of 5.7 million (3.0% of the population) in 1985 (3).
- Between 1997 and 1998 DAWN reported increases in the use of oxycodone (93%), alprazolam (33%), and doxepin (22%) and large decreases in the use of inhalants/solvents/aerosols (23%), methamphetamine/speed (20%), phenobarbital (15%), chlordiazepoxide (13%), and marijuana/hashish (12%) (1).
- An estimated 2.3 million persons first used marijuana in 1998, which corresponds to about 6,000 new users per day (3).
- Between 1997 and 1998 there was no change in the proportion of youth ages 12–17 reporting great risk from using cigarettes, marijuana, cocaine, or alcohol nor was there change in perceptions of ease of obtaining marijuana (56%) or heroin (21%) (3).

■ SOCIETAL COST

Hysteria was the most discussed psychiatric problem of the nineteenth century, but, with their vast impact on our culture and society, SUDs may well become the main challenge for psychiatry and society in the twenty-first century. Not only are they the primary public health problem, SUDs also greatly affect the economic, political, and social fabric of the nation. Measures of the problem include per capita consumption, lifetime and point prevalence, morbidity and mortality, fetal effects of drugs, health care costs, and total cost of lost work time. The monetary cost to the nation is estimated to be greater than $275 billion annually including the related aspects of crime, absenteeism, and treatment (6). Also, 30%–55% of those with mental illness have an SUD (4), which increases the cost of treating primary mental illness.

■ ALCOHOL

- At least 9 million Americans are alcohol dependent and 6 million abuse alcohol.
- The ECA study stated that 13.8% of Americans will have an alcohol-related SUD in their life (4).
- The current yearly costs attributed to alcohol are $166.5 billion, almost double that of the late 1980s (6).
- The rate of frequent drinking among pregnant women, even when controlled for social characteristics, was approximately 4 times higher in 1995 than in 1991 (3.5% in 1995 and 0.8% in 1991) (7).
- Alcohol is a risk factor for violence; nearly 50% of violent deaths are linked with alcohol (8).
- The proportion of alcohol-related deaths was 38.4% in 1998 and 38.5% in 1997 (9).
- Although consumption of alcoholic beverages is illegal for those under age 21, 10.4 million current drinkers were ages 12–20 in 1999 (3). Of this group, 6.8 million engaged in binge drinking, including 2.1 million who would also be classified as heavy drinkers. There have been no statistically significant changes in the rates of underage drinking since 1994.

Morbidity and mortality secondary to alcohol depend on the culture to which the user belongs. The average American over age 14 consumes 2.77 gallons of absolute alcohol annually, which is less than in Russia, France, Scandinavia, and Ireland, but more than in Islamic and Mediterranean cultures or China. In the United

States, approximately one-tenth of those who drink consume half the alcohol sold.

With suicide ranked as the eighth leading cause of death in 1998 and liver disease as the tenth (10), the estimate that 100,000 deaths per year are alcohol related is of importance. The suicide rate for people with alcoholism is 5%–6%, which is much higher than that of the general population (10). Alcoholism is the leading associated factor for cirrhosis even though fewer than 10% of alcoholics develop cirrhosis. There is a high association between alcohol and/or drug use, abuse, addiction, violent crime, and accidents. About 25% of general hospital admissions involve patients with problems related to chronic alcohol use, such as cirrhosis or cardiomyopathy, or related to withdrawal (e.g., seizures, pneumonia, liver failure, and subdural hematomas).

■ COCAINE

- In 1999 an estimated 1.5 million Americans were current cocaine users (3).
- The estimated number of current crack cocaine users was 413,000 in 1999, similar to the number in 1988 (3).
- The highest current cocaine use in 1998 was for people ages 18–25 (3).
- Rates of current cocaine use were 1.3% for blacks, 1.3% for Hispanics, and 0.7% for whites in 1998. Cocaine use increased significantly among Hispanics from 1997 to 1998, from 0.8% to 1.3% (3).
- Men use cocaine more than women (current use in 1998 was 1.1% and 0.5%, respectively) (3).
- Cocaine use is strongly tied to education. Among adults age 18 and older in 1998, the current use rate was 1.4% for those who had not completed high school, 0.8% among high school graduates, 0.7% among those with some college, and 0.5% among college graduates (3).
- Cocaine use is highest among the unemployed: 3.4% of unemployed adults (age 18 and older) were current cocaine users

in 1998, compared with only 0.9% of full-time employed adults and 0.5% of part-time employed adults. However, in absolute terms, of the 1.6 million adult current cocaine users in 1998, 1.1 million (7.0%) were employed either full- or part-time (3).

Although the epidemic use of cocaine in the 1980s abated around 1990, from 1991 to 1997 there was a significant increase in use (3). Increased marketing pressures, lower prices, and availability of more potent, fast-acting cocaine derivatives that can be smoked or used intravenously (e.g., "crack") have increased experimentation, availability, and prevalence of dependence. Interestingly, in the 1970s, experimentation with cocaine was considered relatively safe by many young people and was thought by some experts to be not very dangerous. Cocaine psychosis was rarely reported; lower dosages of cocaine were used and reports of major complications were rare. Since the 1980s, increased market demand has been accompanied by increased availability of purer, more potent forms at lower prices and with more rapid routes of administration, contributing to more frequent severe complications, telescoping of the course of disease progression, and wider problems across social class and race. In adolescent cocaine abusers, the course of progression from use to addiction is much shorter (1.5 years) than it is in adults (4 years).

■ AMPHETAMINES

- From 1991 to 1994 the number of deaths related to methamphetamine use nearly tripled from 151 to 433, and most of those who died were ages 26–44 years (66%), male (80%), and white (80%). Nearly all deaths involved at least one other drug, most often alcohol (30%), heroin (23%), or cocaine (21%) (1).
- Methamphetamine-related emergency department episodes more than tripled, from 4,900 in 1991 to 17,400 in 1994 (11).
- The estimated number of persons who have tried methamphetamine is 4.7 million (3).

The diversion and abuse of amphetamines, which are often prescribed in the treatment of narcolepsy, weight disorders, and depressive disorders, peaked in the 1960s. With better control, legal use, diversion, and illegal use declined. Yet, a substantial increase in use occurred in the 1990s, especially in California. There was an increase in amphetamine-related admissions to publicly funded treatment programs, from 14,000 in 1992 to 53,000 in 1997 (3).

■ OPIOIDS

- Lifetime heroin use prevalence estimates ranged from 2.3 million in 1979 to 1.7 million in 1992, 2 million in 1997, and 2.4 million in 1998 (3).
- An estimated 149,000 persons used heroin for the first time in 1999. The rate of initiation for youths from 1994 to 1999 is at the highest level since the early 1970s (3).
- The estimated number of current heroin users was 68,000 in 1993, 117,000 in 1994, 196,000 in 1995, 216,000 in 1996, 325,000 in 1997, 130,000 in 1998, and 200,000 in 1999 (3).
- Among lifetime heroin users, the proportion who had ever smoked, sniffed, or snorted heroin increased from 55% in 1994 to 75% in 1998, yet, at the same time, the proportion who had ever used heroin with a needle remained relatively unchanged (49% in 1994 and 54% in 1998). This trend toward snorting of heroin is evident among abusers entering publicly funded treatment programs (3).
- The ECA study showed that the use of opioids was greater in males than in females, the ratio being between 3:1 and 4:1 (4).

It is difficult to obtain accurate data on opioid use; estimates come from overdose reports, surveys, prevalence of medical complications, arrests, and treatment program admissions. Heroin abuse is usually a problem in males in urban areas and in those ages 18–25 (3). A higher incidence of nonmedical use of opioids other than heroin is found among whites (12% vs. 7% for minorities) (3).

Minorities have twice the number of heroin abusers as the general population; however, these data may be skewed because whites account for fewer admissions to public facilities and because there may be many white middle-class addicts who do not respond to surveys. When an individual is addicted and part of a cultural group in which heroin use is less endemic, he or she is more likely to have more psychopathology.

Most methadone programs lack adequate availability of treatment openings and lack the capacity for intensive treatment, including enough individual and group counseling, a team approach, and the increasingly important medical and psychiatric support. Unfortunately, most people with psychoactive SUDs, including narcotics addicts, are not in treatment.

■ TOBACCO

- In the United States, cigarette smoking is the leading cause of preventable morbidity and mortality and results in approximately 430,000 deaths each year (12).
- In 1999 an estimated 30.2% of Americans (66.8 million persons) used cigarettes, which is more than in 1998 (27.7%, 60 million) (3).
- The percentage of adults ages 18–25 who smoked rose from 34.6% in 1994 to 41.6% in 1998 and was 39.7% in 1999 (3).
- In 1997, 2.1 million Americans began smoking cigarettes. More than half were younger than age 18, which translates to more than 3,000 new youth smokers per day (3).
- In 1999, 70.4% of all students reported lifetime smoking (13). An estimated 18.2% of youths ages 12–17, or 4.1 million, were current cigarette smokers in 1998 (3).
- In 1999 youths ages 12–17 who currently smoked cigarettes were 7.3 times more likely to use illicit drugs and 16 times more likely to drink heavily than nonsmoking youths (3).
- Prevalence of current smoking in 1999 was significantly higher among Native Americans/Alaska natives (43.1%) than among

most other groups including non-Hispanic blacks (26.6%), and it was higher among non-Hispanic whites (31.9%) than among Hispanics (24.4%) or Asians/Pacific Islanders (18.6%) (3).

- Current smoking rates are highest among persons with 9–11 years of education (35.4%) and lowest among those with 16 years of education (11.6%). The rate is higher for persons living below the poverty level (33.3%) than among those at or above that level (24.6%) (3).

Although cigarette use has been decreasing among men, it has been increasing among women. Educational campaigns, self-help groups, self-help literature, treatment facilities, and government legislation have been aimed at decreasing the numbers of smokers. Smoking in public places (e.g., restaurants, airplanes, hospitals, and work environments) is increasingly restricted, and the rights of non-smokers are being considered.

■ PHENCYCLIDINE AND KETAMINE

In certain eastern areas of the United States, phencyclidine (also called PCP or "angel dust") abuse is epidemic and is frequently associated with violent and bizarre behavior. Its use had reached a nadir, but it has become more popular again. Ketamine abuse has also risen (3).

■ HALLUCINOGENS

- There were an estimated 1.2 million new users of hallucinogens in 1999. From 1992 to 1996 the initiation rate among potential new youth users ages 12–17 increased from 14.5 to 29.5 per thousand; the initiation rate was essentially constant from 1996 to 1999 (3).
- The rate of current use of hallucinogens was 0.4% in 1999 (3).

Lysergic acid diethylamide (LSD) achieved its greatest popularity in the 1960s and 1970s but has once again become popular in some high school communities. Some students have discovered that LSD is not easily detectable in urine samples. In the 1960s psychedelic drugs were romanticized as part of a cultural movement that included a style of mind expansion and poetic expression in rock culture, and they became associated with turning away from war, rebelling against society, and "dropping out." Southwestern Native Americans had long used psilocybin 21 in religious ceremonies. Although there have been few designer drugs of the indolealkylamine derivative type, of which LSD is one, there is a steady flow of new (designer) phenylalkylamine derivatives, including the ring-substituted amphetamines such as MDA, MDMA (ecstasy, old and new), and MDEA. Ecstasy first appeared at "raves," but it has grown in popularity and has been increasingly implicated in some deaths. There are 12 known natural hallucinogens but more than 100 synthetics to date.

■ MARIJUANA

- First use of marijuana in the United States was estimated at 2.3 million in 1999 (3).
- Frequent users were estimated at 6.8 million in 1998; this is significantly more than in 1995 (5.3 million) (3).
- In 1999 approximately 75% of current illicit drug users were marijuana/hashish users (3).
- The prevalence of current marijuana use among youths more than doubled from 1992 to 1995, from 3.4% to 8.2%. About 1 in 12 youths ages 12–17 (8.3%) was a current marijuana user in 1998 (3).
- Among females, the age of first use has been declining, and the prevalence of secondary problems has been rising (14).

Worldwide, cannabis may be the most widely abused illicit substance of all; in the United States it accounts for 75% of all illicit drug use (3). Trends and demographic differences are generally similar for marijuana/hashish use and for other illicit drug use. Increased potency of the available cannabis and concomitant heavy use have led to an increase in medical and psychological risk. Marijuana use peaked among adolescents in the 1970s; however, it continues to be a gateway drug for other substances. Compassionate use of medical marijuana for chronic and debilitating disease has been supported by an Institute of Medicine report (15).

■ INHALANTS

Inhalant use stabilized in 1996 after 4 years of increase, according to the National High School Senior and Young Adult Survey (16). Fortunately, annual prevalence has decreased between grades 8 and 12 as the view that inhalants are dangerous increased. Inhalants tend to be used by males 13–15 years old in difficult socioeconomic circumstances and by those in certain subcultures (e.g., Native Americans from the United States and Mexico). Inhalant intoxication has been closely associated with aggressive, disruptive, antisocial behavior and is also associated with poor performance in school, increased family disruption, and other drug abuse (3).

■ SEDATIVES, HYPNOTICS, AND ANXIOLYTICS

Since 1976 there has been a decline in abuse of benzodiazepines and sedative hypnotics, but these useful drugs still have potential for abuse. Their abuse is related to the high prevalence of anxiety disorders. Approximately 1 user in 5 abuses sedatives; this abuse may be iatrogenic or the result of diverted supplies. Barbiturate overdoses, once frequently the cause of emergency room visits, have decreased because of the decreasing popularity of barbiturate prescription and use. They have been largely replaced by benzodiazepines, which have a higher index of therapeutic safety, including a smaller chance of causing respiratory depression.

Still, physicians prescribing benzodiazepines and barbiturates need to be aware of the potential for abuse, especially by individuals with risk factors of alcohol and drug abuse. It is difficult to determine incidence and prevalence of alcoholism and other drug abuse because of a lack of clear criteria for diagnosis of dependence, the variety of subpopulations studied, the tolerance of a particular subculture for drug-related behaviors, and dishonesty associated with reporting substance use problems.

■ POLYSUBSTANCE PROBLEMS

- In the ECA study data, 30% of alcoholics also met criteria for abuse of or dependence on other substances (4).
- In the ECA study the most common comorbidity with an SUD was another SUD, nicotine dependence, which may have effects on treatment of a patient's psychiatric conditions, and/or EPS (4).
- The ECA study provided odds ratios for SUDs among populations with certain psychopathologies: major depressive disorder, 2:1; panic disorder, 3:1; schizophrenia, 5:1; and bipolar disorder, 7:1 (4).

Recently, polysubstance abuse has increased, with combined use of alcohol, heroin, cocaine, methadone, and tobacco. Combinations of used substances have been especially noted in young and female patients. Teenagers tend to progress from alcohol and tobacco use to marijuana use and use of barbiturates, codeine, or other opioids before abusing heroin. Deaths related to overdose are more commonly associated with combinations of alcohol, depressants, and heroin than with cocaine, which has recently received greater public attention. Of note, treatment for abuse of one substance usually has the effect of reducing use of others (e.g., a methadone maintenance program reduces comorbid cocaine abuse) (3).

■ UNDERLYING ISSUES AFFECTING ADDICTION MAGNITUDE

Medical and Psychiatric Complications

Medical and psychiatric problems, including the effects of intoxication, overdose, and withdrawal, and the consequences of chronic use associated with SUDs produce morbidity and mortality. All organ systems are affected by SUDs. The following syndromes are among the major complications: gastritis, ulcers, pancreatitis, liver disease, cardiomyopathy, anemia, neurological complications, sexual dysfunction, fetal alcohol syndrome, and renal failure. Increased rates of oropharyngeal, esophageal, and hepatic cancer have been reported. Delirium tremens, intoxication, and other withdrawal syndromes can lead to death. The use of unsterile needles contributes to the spread of AIDS, hepatitis, skin abscesses, endocarditis, mycotic aneurysms, septic arthritis, osteomyelitis, meningitis, and lung abscesses. And, not least, suicide remains a great complication of substance abuse.

AIDS and Intravenous Drugs

The intravenous use of opioids and cocaine has been a major risk factor in the spread of AIDS through needle sharing and disinhibition of risk-taking behavior. The latter includes promiscuous and unsafe sexual behavior. HIV-positive female addicts and sexual partners of addicts who are HIV positive have the added risk of spreading AIDS to fetuses. Addicts vary widely regarding their rates of HIV infection and, for those who are infected, stage of AIDS. The urban poor and minorities are the hardest hit by intravenous needle sharing. When heroin addicts who are on a methadone maintenance program continue intravenous cocaine use, reduction of the spread of HIV is more difficult, even when there is relatively high methadone compliance. Happily, by the end of the 1990s, with the newest antiretroviral medications, there was evidence for a decline in prevalence and a lower incidence of HIV contracted by intravenous drug users (17).

Factors Contributing to Complications

Poor self-care, dietary problems, the use of unsterile needles, the admixture of unknown quantities of impure substances in the abused drug, and the psychosocial problems associated with addiction (e.g., the increased personal risk of crime, suicidality, and homicidality) contribute to the medical and dental complications of drug abuse and must be added to the effects of the drug itself. The additional use of alcohol can further contribute to liver failure in those addicted to intravenous drugs who also have hepatitis, and it may lower resistance to infections and increase the incidence of lung diseases (e.g., pneumonia and tuberculosis). Renal disease may be caused by antigen-antibody immune complexes resulting from infection and by hypertension, which frequently accompanies substance abuse, especially alcohol and stimulant abuse. Cocaine use may contribute to hypertension, tachycardia, and arrhythmia and is a cause of sudden death. Patients with combinations of problems (e.g., alcohol withdrawal, diabetes, and hypertension) who are given antidepressants may be at especially high risk for cardiac arrhythmias, vascular problems, and sudden death. Chronic substance use can reduce sexual performance and desire in both sexes. Studies indicate that marijuana use as well as chronic alcohol use decreases serum testosterone in males. Poor nutrition and vitamin deficiencies contribute to low resistance to illness.

Denial and Stigma

The patient with SUDs may demonstrate denial, dissimulation, and memory problems related to organicity, as well as a fear of stigmatization, making it difficult to obtain a clear history. Either because of refusal to cooperate or as a result of being socially isolated, the patient may not have family or friends who can be interviewed. Due to intoxication or overdose, the patient may be unable to answer coherently. Often the patient who is seeking help has been coerced into seeing a doctor by family, an employer, the court, or a family physician and has mixed feelings about cooperating. In addition to the possibility of a long-term disrespect for authority figures, which may stem from being a child of an alcoholic, the patient may have had bad experiences with physicians who were not well informed about SUDs. The patient needs reassurance that there is reason to be hopeful about the outcome of treatment, and an effort needs to be made to reduce blame and guilt. What the patient does not tell the doctor may be as important as what the patient does say; an alert clinician must watch for observable signs, symptoms, and mental status characterized by high denial, projection, and rationalization.

Facility Prejudices

Patients who are mentally ill and have SUDs are often inadequately managed in general psychiatric facilities and in free-standing alcohol and drug rehabilitation facilities that do not provide integrated treatment for patients with dual diagnosis. Minimal contact with the psychiatric consultant and primary treatment by alcoholism counselors, who may have insufficient psychiatric training, can lead to underdiagnosis and insufficient treatment of additional psychiatric problems. For patients with psychosis, an abstinence-oriented program needs to be flexible even when relapses occur. Many psychiatric halfway houses do not accept alcoholics, and halfway houses for substance abusers often do not accept patients on medications. Confrontational methods that are useful in therapeutic communities and self-help groups may be detrimental to those with more severe psychiatric illness. The full-service facilities with psychiatric treatment and rehabilitation are expensive; however, they represent a healthy integration of treatment approaches.

Managed Care

The need to reduce health care costs has driven great change in the practice of medicine in the United States since the late 1980s. This has had an impact on the care of patients with SUDs. The trend has indeed driven a number of clinical changes including the forging of health care systems that attempt to save money by coordinating care and reducing unnecessary spending or interventions. The emphasis is on outpatient care, including outpatient detoxification. In recent years managed care has reduced the amount spent on addiction treatment by 75%, and many of the cuts have been detrimental to good care. It is hoped that more resources can be marshaled in the future for addiction treatment in public, private, and prison settings.

The Internet

The rise of the Internet has provided a tool with which those who abuse drugs can obtain information about drugs of abuse, including how to get them, how to hide them, how to grow plants, who to buy from and who not to buy from, and where the interdiction agencies are concentrating their energies and attention. Most importantly, both illicit and controlled substances are sold over the Internet. This medium connects many people—some of whom may have nefarious purposes. Yet other information and connections gained over the Internet can be of great help, and Table 2–1 includes such sites.

TABLE 2–1. **Helpful Internet sites**

American Psychiatric Association	www.psych.org
National Institute on Drug Abuse	www.drugabuse.gov
SAMHSA (includes NHS and DAWN)	www.samhsa.gov
Monitoring the Future Survey	www.monitoringthefuture.org
National Center for Health Statistics/CDC/MMWR	www.cdc.gov/nchs/default.htm
National Comorbidity Survey	www.hcp.med.harvard.edu/ncs
Addiction Resource Guide	www.addictionresourceguide.com
Office of National Drug Control Policy	www.whitehousedrugpolicy.gov
Silver Hill Hospital	www.silverhillhospital.com
McLean Hospital	www.mcleanhospital.org
Northwestern Medical Center	www.nums.nwu.edu/psychiatry
Sheppard Pratt Health System	www.sheppardpratt.org
Betty Ford Center	www.bettyfordcenter.org
Hazelden Foundation	www.hazelden.org/index.cfm
American Academy of Addiction Psychiatry	www.aaap.org

■ REFERENCES

1. Office of Applied Studies: Drug Abuse Warning Network, Annual Medical Examiner Data, 1998. Rockville, MD, Substance Abuse and Mental Health Services Administration, 2000

2. Johnston LD, O'Malley PM, Bachman JG: The Monitoring the Future National Survey Results on Adolescent Drug Use: Overview of Key Findings, 1999 (NIH Publication 00-4690). Rockville, MD, National Institute on Drug Abuse, 2000

3. Office of Applied Studies: National Household Survey on Drug Abuse. Rockville, MD, Substance Abuse and Mental Health Services Administration, 2000

4. Regier DA, Farmer ME, Rae DS, et al: Co-morbidity of mental disorders with alcohol and other drug abuse: results from the Epidemiologic Catchment Area study. JAMA 264:2511–2518, 1990

5. Kessler RC, Crum RM, Warner LA, et al: Lifetime co-occurrence of DSM-III-R alcohol abuse and dependence with other psychiatric disorders in the National Comorbidity Survey. Arch Gen Psychiatry 54:313–321, 1997

6. Harwood H, Fountain D, Livermore G, et al: The Economic Costs of Alcohol and Drug Abuse in the United States, 1992. Washington, DC, National Institute on Drug Abuse and National Institute on Alcohol Abuse and Alcoholism, 1998

7. Alcohol consumption among pregnant and childbearing-aged women: United States, 1991 and 1995. MMWR 46:346–350, 1997

8. The Role of Co-Occurring Substance Abuse and Mental Illness in Violence: Workshop Summary Division of Neuroscience and Behavioral Health, Institute of Medicine. Washington, DC, National Academy Press, 1999

9. Alcohol involvement in fatal motor-vehicle crashes: United States, 1997–1998. MMWR 48:1086–1087, 1999

10. Murphy SL: Deaths: Final Data for 1998 (National Vital Statistics Reports, Vol 48, No 11). Hyattsville, MD, National Center for Vital Statistics, 2000

11. Increasing morbidity and mortality associated with abuse of methamphetamine: United States, 1991–1994. MMWR 44:882–886, 1995

12. Cigarette smoking among adults: United States, 1997. MMWR 48:993–996, 1999

13. Trends in cigarette smoking among high school students: United States, 1991–1999. MMWR 49:755–758, 2000

14. Greenfield SF, O'Leary G: Sex differences in marijuana use in the United States. Harvard Review of Psychiatry 6:297–303, 1999

15. Division of Neuroscience and Behavioral Health, Institute of Medicine: Marijuana and Medicine: Assessing the Science Base. Edited by Joy JE, Watson SJ Jr, Benson JA Jr. Washington, DC, National Academy Press, 1999

16. Johnston LD, O'Malley PM, Bachman JG: National annual high school senior and young adult survey. Washington, DC, U.S. Government Printing Office, 1997

17. Des Jarlias DC, Marmor M, Friedman P, et al: HIV incidence among injection drug users in New York City, 1992–1997: evidence for a declining epidemic. Am J Public Health 90: 352–359, 2000

3

DEVELOPMENTAL
ISSUES IN THE FIELD

■ THE DISEASE CONCEPT

The validity of disorders involving substance use has been challenged more than the validity of any other category of disorders. Some critics have reductionistically asserted that substance abuse is simply a moral problem, and therefore, choosing to abuse a substance is a decision that deserves shame and punishment more than empathy and treatment. Others assume addiction is simply excessive or compulsive use of a substance. In contrast, the concept of addiction as a disease may focus on the addict's lack of stability, lack of perfect health, discomfort, difference from the norm, discernible biological components that predispose to addiction, or response to biological treatment; definitions can be narrow or broad, can be culturally defined, and can change over time. Three (probably intertwined) aspects of addiction are increasingly seen as central to its understanding: addiction is the compulsion to use the substance, addiction is a brain disease, and addiction is a chronic medical disorder.

Defining addiction as a compulsion means that the individual uses the substance at all costs, even in the face of severe negative consequences. As described below, the evidence that there is a biological component to addiction is growing. The existence of biological markers provides a basis for genetic vulnerability to abuse particular substances. Furthermore, research is being focused on the long-term changes in synaptic architecture and alterations in neurotransmitter physiology that may show that the brain of the addicted patient is different as a result of excessive use—a difference that creates and maintains the compulsion to use (1). By no means should the perspective that addiction has a biological basis diminish the social, environmental, or personal aspects of addiction. However, biological evidence is important because, at the least, it lends support to the disease model of addiction.

Another development in the conceptualization of addiction regards the nature of the disease. Addictions have chronic courses, and abstinence is often punctuated with multiple relapses. The individual abuser suffers not only from complications of use but also from social and economic problems that result from abuse. More and more of those involved in the treatment of addiction have compared substance use disorders (SUDs) to other chronic medical disorders such as diabetes mellitus, arthritis, or asthma—diseases that we can treat but perhaps never entirely cure—and in which relapses, especially those related to choices patients make, are to be expected. In this view the influence of returning to the environment in which the former cocaine abuser used is analogous to the smoky room that causes the child with asthma to have an attack (2).

One implication of this view is that society's moralizing about substance abuse has had, for generations, the effect of impeding the recognition of SUDs, which in turn has resulted in a lack of research on these disorders and a lack of appropriate care for those affected. If society can be rid of the concept of substance dependence and abuse as the fault of the individual, greater emphasis could be placed on treatment rather than punishment. This could lead to reduction of overly harsh sentencing, such as the Rockefeller laws in New York State, and the use of drug courts and alternatives to sentencing that emphasize treatment for nonviolent drug crimes. On the other hand, the concept of SUDs as medical conditions and not the fault of the individual could be misconstrued to imply that abuse, dependence, or even relapse are acceptable and that abstinence is irrelevant, which could be used to support legalization of drug use. Most addiction and legal experts are against legalization because they believe it would lead to increased substance availability, increased craving, and increased prevalence and complications of addictions.

Nosology

Since the 1960s, American psychiatrists have become increasingly interested in refining the classification of disorders, with the hope that further refinement will lead to the discovery of valid, distinct diseases. This interest continues in the DSM-IV era. DSM-IV and its Text Revision, DSM-IV-TR (3), direct the diagnostician to differentiate between alcohol dependencies with physiological components and those without. A study of 3,395 people dependent on alcohol suggested that physical dependence, especially marked by withdrawal, predicts a more severe course of alcoholism (4).

■ NEUROBIOLOGY OF ADDICTIONS: CLINICAL IMPLICATIONS OF RESEARCH FINDINGS

Genetics: Familial Studies and High-Risk Populations

Fifty years ago, Jellinek and Jolliffee established that alcoholism occurs in families. Although genetic influences in alcoholism and other drug abuse patterns in both men and women have become fairly well established through twin, adoption, and split sibling studies, neither the mode of transmission nor the nature of what is being transmitted is clear. Some studies have suggested that, with regard to alcohol abuse, tolerance is the transmitted trait. In establishing the genetic bases of cocaine and cannabis abuse, other studies have proposed that a general vulnerability to a particular substance is transmitted and that the affected person might become addicted after only one exposure (5).

Further lines of research in the genetics of addiction, including pharmacogenetics and gender differences in genetic transmission, will address variability among patients. A greater understanding of genetics could lead to better efforts to prevent addiction, and an understanding of the pathogenesis of addiction could lead to new treatments.

Biological Markers

Biological markers are associated findings, if not causal findings, that may help us to identify high-risk individuals before the onset of abuse, identify dependence when it does exist, and follow the course of the disease (see Chapter 6, Laboratory Findings and Diagnostic Instruments).

Identifying children at high risk for alcoholism or substance abuse has been one major research thrust. Schuckit has been working on multiple markers in biological sons of alcoholics (6) (Table 3–1). His results have included positive findings of decreased subjective feelings of intoxication in not-yet-alcoholic children of alcoholics and of less impairment of motor performance. He has also reported less body sway or static ataxia with alcohol challenge and less change in cortisol and prolactin levels when compared to controls. Schuckit has been attempting to determine the predictive value of these markers. The clinician who is working with adolescent or young adult populations especially should focus closely on the patient's initial experiences with alcohol. Does the adolescent drink much more than his or her peers and not show signs or symptoms of intoxication? What is the best advice for a young person who drinks and experiences few adverse effects in the beginning but has a strong family history of dependence? An early choice of abstinence may be the safest form of prevention for these individuals. Often these teenagers describe their first real experience with alcohol as a revelation—an ''ah ha'' experience—in which alcohol

---

TABLE 3–1. **Possible markers of alcoholism in biological sons of alcoholics**

Decreased subjective feelings of intoxication
Less impairment of motor performance
Less body sway
Less static ataxia
Less change in cortisol and prolactin findings
Low P300 amplitude (electroencephalogram)
Increased alpha-wave activity

---

is discovered as an acceptable way to handle anxiety, decrease stress, and express emotions.

Electroencephalographic Markers

A finding among abstinent alcoholics and sons of alcoholics is an alteration of normal auditory brain stem potentials. The P300 event-related potential (ERP) (the voltage of the third positive electro-encephalogram wave in response to this stimulus) is of low amplitude in alcoholics and abstinent young sons of alcoholic men. The P300 component may be related to motivational properties of stimuli and involved in the process of memory. The association with alcoholism is well replicated, but the finding is not limited to alcoholics or their children. Thus although specificity of this possible marker is not high enough for predictive value, this is a promising area of research. Increased alpha-wave activity with alcohol exposure in alcoholics compared with nonalcoholic subjects has also been reported (Table 3–1). These findings might be more valid for visual stimuli than for auditory stimuli (7). These studies may reflect brain stem demyelination.

Alcohol Metabolism

Alcohol dehydrogenase and aldehyde dehydrogenase are the two hepatic enzymes involved in the metabolism of ethanol. Current studies have been undertaken to learn how the five genes that make up alcohol dehydrogenase and are transmitted on the long arm of chromosome 4 could be correlated with the threefold variability that is known to exist in ethanol metabolism among humans.

Neurochemical Markers

There has been controversy over whether there is low activity of platelet monoamine oxidase B (MAO B) in alcoholics. Low activity may be even more apparent in Type II than in Type I alcoholics and persists despite abstinence. However, it may be more a marker of state than a trait. Adenylate cyclase in platelets and lymphocytes has also been studied, and its level is usually reduced in alcoholics, but the significance of this is unknown.

Flushing Response

The flushing response occurs in Asian populations and is the result of a single point mutation. It may protect an individual from excessive alcohol intake. In some cultures, it reduces drinking, in others, such as among Koreans, it does not.

Neuropsychological Performance

Prospective longitudinal studies of sons of alcoholics have reported some evidence of poor neuropsychological performance in areas such as categorizing ability, organization, planning, abstracting, and problem-solving ability. Tarter and Edwards suggested that minimal brain dysfunction or conduct disorder may predispose an individual toward alcoholism and may be an expression of an underlying inherited temperament (8). Risk-taking, sensation-seeking individuals are thought to be at high risk.

■ CELLULAR PATHOPHYSIOLOGY OF ADDICTION

Advances in cellular and molecular biology have been staggering over the past decade, and this is no less the case in psychiatry and addiction research. There is increasing evidence that craving and addiction to virtually all abused substances are related to the dopaminergic systems in the brain, especially the mesolimbic reward system and the areas to which it projects: the limbic system and the orbitofrontal cortex (9). This relationship between addiction and the dopaminergic systems has even been seen in the case of cannabinoids (10), and it may result not only from homeostatic adaptations of neurons, but also from the neural plasticity and synaptic rearrangement that is the consequence of activation of particular signal transduction pathways between the stimulus and the resulting gene expression. The idea is that addiction is not just a degenerative disease or a lesion but a learned process in which long-term memory occurs (inappropriately) at the molecular level. Such a view reduces the serious nature of relapse (2). It will be necessary in the future to study mechanisms of molecular memory and their relation to decreases in addiction.

As noted above, there is evidence that the compulsion to use particular substances is the result of craving that is the consequence of an environmental cue. Compulsion is at least partly seated in the mesolimbic system.

■ PREVENTION EFFORTS

Role of Prevention

With greater scientific advances in the understanding of alcoholism and other addictions in terms of description, etiology, pathogenesis, course, and epidemiology, there is an increasing possibility that strategies for prevention may be successful. Advances in genetic understanding of familial alcoholism, for example, may lead to discovery of genetic markers that can identify a high-risk population. However, psychiatrists and other health professionals are still far from being able to match prevention of infectious disease by vaccination and prevention of parasitic disease by improved sanitary and public health measures. Efforts to improve border control, improve social planning in law enforcement, and increase public information have not led to major changes in the magnitude of the problem. The vast cost of addiction requires greater research to develop a better understanding of the illness, its prevention, and its treatment.

Educational Programs

Primary prevention efforts have focused heavily on school-based and work-based alcohol education programs and mass media campaigns, as well as attempts to limit availability of the agent. Programs targeted at students, parents, and employees have significantly increased knowledge regarding alcohol and other substance abuse. However, it is harder to achieve changes in attitudes toward alcohol and drugs, and changes in drinking behavior have been modest or difficult to demonstrate.

Efforts at life-skills training that focus on values clarification abilities, decision making, and drug refusal may be more effective in changing attitudes than are cognitive interventions aimed at increasing knowledge alone. Based on social learning theory, programs teach young people how to refuse drugs and provide information about the hazards of drugs, peer pressure, and expanding one's specific behavioral repertoire for saying no. Through rehearsal of a variety of rejecting responses, it is hoped that in the appropriate situation these responses will be available. Such programs often begin in middle school (usually from sixth to ninth grade) and use peer leaders to enhance social resistance skills based on improved self-management and self-efficacy. The factors that increase adolescent substance abuse include peer pressure, role modeling, desire to obtain adult status, curiosity, low self-esteem, and an unstable family. Drugs may be used to solve painful affects, initiate sexual intimacy, and promote greater group identification. Student assistance model programs include the following: education and groups, with children of alcoholics especially targeted; treatment or referral for students who abuse; early screening of students with behavioral changes; and work with parents and community groups.

Adolescents frequently experiment with alcohol and drug use. A national program of teaching children to refuse substances has been successful only in part. Because of the ubiquitous presence of alcohol in our culture, coming to personal terms with alcohol and drug abuse may represent a developmental task for some teenagers. A ''just say no'' approach may be most important for those at highest risk for developing an alcohol problem, such as children of alcoholics. Most educational programs touch on myths about alcohol, alcohol advertisement, causes of alcoholism, and the effects of alcohol and drugs on life satisfaction and also instill positive social skills and behaviors.

12-Step and Other Self-Help Programs

Self-help groups such as Alateen, Al-Anon, Alcoholics Anonymous, Adult Children of Alcoholics, and Mothers Against Drunk Driving provide support for alcoholics and those affected by alcoholics. These groups also disseminate educational materials, help distribute information, and, indirectly through 12-step work, aid at early case finding and intervention. Some groups supply important lobbying power.

Mass Media

Mass media prevention campaigns on radio and television and through the press use messages delivered by popular peer models, prominent sports figures, celebrities, or parental role models (e.g., Nancy Reagan, Rosalyn Carter, Betty Ford, and Tipper Gore). An active public service announcement campaign of donated advertising time produced by Partnership for a Drug Free America (which has been supplemented with federal financing) has been very effective in changing attitudes, challenging myths, and promoting increased communication between parents and children about drugs. Between 1997 and 1999 illicit substance use among adolescents (ages 12–17) significantly declined, perhaps as a result of this program. This effort in part counters advertisers' use of mass media to increase sales of addictive substances (e.g., alcohol and tobacco). Use and abuse of psychoactive substances are frequently glamorized on television and in films. Commercials that portray alcohol positively, with images including camaraderie, relaxation, and enjoyment, contain important subliminal messages, although it is not clear what negative impact this advertising has on prevention efforts. Alcohol-containing products such as wine coolers, frequently packaged to look like soft drinks, are sold over the counter in grocery stores and are designed to appeal to a youth market.

Prevention at the Workplace

The high loss of employee productivity associated with intoxication and chronic substance abuse can lead to safety hazards, illness, absenteeism, poor work quality, and bad morale. Preemployment drug screens are now used routinely in the National Football League, in major league baseball, and in hockey leagues. Use of drug screens at the workplace has raised ethical issues such as the individual's right to privacy versus prevention and treatment for the good of the group. Olympic athletes are required to give urine samples before events. Abuse of steroids has led to broken dreams and questions about unfair competition. Increasingly, society is demanding use of drug screens, especially in jobs for which hazards produced by impairment are high (e.g., airline pilots, surgeons, transportation workers).

When management and unions work together with employee assistance professionals and have clear policies that are well known to all concerned, confrontation techniques are especially effective. Employees are offered treatment and rehabilitation, with progressive job action taken if the employee continues to have difficulty functioning at work. Additional disciplinary measures can often be avoided if confrontation occurs early enough; also, good employee assistance programs have high numbers of voluntary participants.

Social Policy and Legal Efforts

Greater availability of addictive substances leads to greater craving for them and use of them. Because alcohol and tobacco are widely available, cheap, and legal, they are the most heavily used. Due to the enormous profits that can be gleaned from the sale of illegal drugs, it has proved to be extremely difficult to limit the influx of illegal substances. Illegal drug use is tied to market value, cost, availability, and quality. Limiting availability of alcohol through price manipulation, outlet availability, hours of sale, and age restriction policies is one strategy to reduce overall consumption. Forbidding grocery stores from selling distilled alcohol and the banning of hotel room refrigeration dispensers are examples of efforts to reduce exposure of recovering alcoholics and teenagers to marketing that increases availability. Overall rates of liver cirrhosis are correlated with alcohol availability and total alcohol consumption and may be reduced by efforts to limit consumption. The legal drinking age has been raised to 21 throughout the nation, and studies indicate that this has decreased motor vehicle accidents and deaths among adolescents. Limiting tobacco advertising and use in public places has been another effective measure in an effort to achieve the surgeon general's goal of a smokeless society. Legal cases against tobacco companies have recently led to large settlements, and it is hoped that some of those monies will be used for further public health efforts. Of note, there is good reason to believe that schizophrenic patients can successfully tolerate smoking cessation programs (11).

High-Risk Groups

Children of Alcoholics

Twin, adoption, and half-sibling genetic studies and studies of familial versus nonfamilial alcoholism indicate that children of alcoholics are at a fourfold higher risk of developing alcoholism. Efforts to target programs for those at high risk for heart disease, obesity, hypertension, and high cholesterol have been paralleled by programs to assist the high-risk group of children of alcoholics to achieve alternative alcohol-free lifestyles. Familial alcoholics have an earlier onset of problem drinking, more severe social consequences, less consistently stable family involvement, poor academic and social performance in school, more antisocial behavior, and poorer prognosis in treatment (Table 3–2).

TABLE 3–2. **Characteristics of familial alcoholics**

Earlier onset of problem drinking
More severe social consequences
Less consistently stable family involvement
Poor academic and social performance in school
More antisocial behavior
Poorer prognosis in treatment

A major movement has grown up around the problem of being an adult child of an alcoholic. Children of alcoholics frequently suffer from stigma, alienation, estrangement, and isolation. Their parents are frequently inconsistent and emotionally depriving, force them into inappropriate roles, and are more likely to be aggressive or sexually abusive, have difficult divorces, and abandon their children. Struggling with feelings of anger, confusion, and helplessness, these children tend to distrust authority figures, depend more on peers, and pick friends from similarly troubled families. Distrust of authority figures is likely to be extended to doctors, nurses, and other health care professionals. These children grow up protesting their parents' behavior, trying to be different, but they often end up having the same problems. This may explain why self-help groups, group therapy, and family approaches that take into account peer support are so successful.

College Students

Despite continued efforts to reduce abuse of alcohol among teens and college students, problems continue. Binge drinking on campuses is rampant. Freshmen are often away from home for the first time and think that drinking and substance experimentation is cool and perhaps will get them into a fraternity or sorority, some of which may foster heavy drinking. One study found that brief intervention as a primary step might be helpful especially if done in a nonjudgmental, practical way (12). Lack of supervision of students by universities and colleges contributes to the problem. Most colleges have inadequate programs for alcohol abuse detection and treatment. Designated driver programs are helpful for harm reduction.

Relationship to Other Prevention Efforts

Early treatment of an alcohol or drug problem may also help prevent development of other problems, such as depression or an antisocial personality. Similarly, early treatment of depression, attention-deficit/hyperactivity disorder, or anxiety disorders may help to prevent the development of an alcohol or drug problem and thereby progression to an antisocial personality. These illnesses have complicated interactions, and each can precede, contribute to, or coexist with the others. Attention-deficit/hyperactivity disorder can be seen as a gateway disorder in which there should be early identification and intervention regarding SUDs.

New cases of HIV infection have finally plateaued, but TB remains rampant. With multidrug-resistant TB, it is all the more important to develop a systematic services approach to protect caregivers and patients alike (13). For HIV in the United States, however, the story has recently taken a positive turn (14). Regardless, the need for patient education and treatment and heightened awareness of infection risks is great.

■ TREATMENT ISSUES

Standardization of Treatment

The American Psychiatric Association's effort to develop practice guidelines (15) has produced a valuable document intended to improve the evaluation and treatment of patients with SUDs. The creators used reviews of the literature to rate treatments. Like DSM, the practice guidelines will need to be revised periodically. Another valuable group of guidelines, the Expert Consensus guidelines, addresses particular clinical situations. Finally, the American Society of Addiction Medicine placement criteria offer clear directions for disposition (16). The clinician should remember never to use these guidelines as cookbooks, but as minimal standards of care.

Differential Therapeutics

Practitioners in the field of SUD treatment continue to attempt to create a differential therapeutics, because all patients are individuals with particular unique problems. There are studies that show that tailoring of treatment is helpful for patients (17). However, the resulting variation often makes it difficult to demonstrate differential treatment outcomes.

Treatment Approaches

The idea that psychotherapy combined with pharmacotherapy is, in the long term, better than either alone has been proven in the treatment of SUDs, for example, in the case of using naltrexone in the treatment of alcohol abuse (18) and in the negative effects of discontinuing methadone maintenance (19). Cognitive-behavioral therapy is an effective treatment for depression in alcoholic patients (20).

Office-Based Treatment

A number of studies have considered the use of opioid replacement treatment in noninstitutional settings. In particular, the use of buprenorphine and methadone has been investigated. The hope is that more people can be treated for opioid addiction. It is important to increase the number of treatment sites because the organized, approved programs in central locations reach only 14% of patients with opioid dependence.

Integrated Services

Patients having dual diagnoses deserve comprehensive, integrated treatment. Outpatient care for such patients must include aggressive outreach, case management, and a longitudinal, stagewise, motivational approach to substance abuse treatment.

■ REFERENCES

1. Leshner AI: Addiction is a brain disease and it matters. Science 278:45–47, 1997

2. O'Brien CP, McLellan AT: Myths about the treatment of addiction. Lancet 347:237–240, 1996

3. American Psychiatric Association: Diagnostic and Statistical Manual of Mental Disorders, 4th Edition, Text Revision. Washington, DC, American Psychiatric Association, 2000

4. Schuckit MA, Smith TL, Daeppen JB, et al: Clinical relevance of the distinction between alcohol dependence with and without a physiological component. Am J Psychiatry 155:733–740, 1998

5. Kendler KS, Prescott CA: Cocaine use, abuse, and dependence in a population-based sample of female twins. Br J Psychiatry 173:345–350, 1998

6. Schuckit MA: Biological vulnerability to alcoholism. J Consult Clin Psychol 55:301–309, 1987

7. Polich J, Bloom FE: P300, alcoholism heritablility, and stimulus modality. Alcohol 17:149–156, 1999

8. Tarter RE, Edwards K: Psychological factors associated with the risk for alcoholism. Alcohol Clin Exp Res 12:471–480, 1988

9. Leshner AI, Koob GF: Drugs of abuse and the brain. Proc Assoc Am Physicians 111:99–108, 1999

10. Diana M, Melis M, Muntoni AL, et al: Mesolimbic dopaminergic decline after cannabinoid withdrawal. Proc Natl Acad Sci U S A 95:10,269–10,273, 1998

11. Addington J, el-Guebaly N, Campbell W, et al: Smoking cessation treatment for patients with schizophrenia. Am J Psychiatry 155:974–976, 1998

12. Marlatt GA, Baer JS, Kivlahan DR, et al: Screening and brief intervention for high-risk college student drinkers: results from a 2-year follow-up assessment. J Consult Clin Psychol 66:604–615, 1998

13. Perlman DC, Saloman N, Perkins MP, et al: Tuberculosis in drug users. Clin Infect Dis 21:1263–1264, 1995

14. Des Jarlias DC, Marmor M, Friedman P, et al: HIV incidence among injection drug users in New York City, 1992–1997: evi-

dence for a declining epidemic. Am J Public Health 90:352–359, 2000

15. Work Group on Substance Use Disorders: Practice guideline for the treatment of patients with substance use disorders: alcohol, cocaine, opioids. Am J Psychiatry 152 (suppl), 1995

16. American Society of Addiction Medicine: Patient placement criteria for the treatment of substance-related disorders, 2nd Edition. Chevy Chase, MD, American Society of Addiction Medicine, 1996

17. Mclellan AT, Grissom GR, Zanis D, et al: Problem-service "matching" in addiction treatment: a prospective study in four programs. Arch Gen Psychiatry 54:730–735, 1997

18. O'Malley SS, Jaffe AJ, Chang G, et al: Six-month follow-up of naltrexone and psychotherapy for alcohol dependence. Arch Gen Psychiatry 53:217–224, 1996

19. Sees KL, Delucci KL, Masson C, et al: Methadone maintenance versus 180-day psychosocially enriched detoxification for treatment of opioid dependence. JAMA 283:1303–1310, 2000

20. Brown RA, Evans DM, Miller IW, et al: CBT for depression in alcoholism. J Consult Clin Psychol 65:715–726, 1997

4

DEFINITION, PRESENTATION, AND DIAGNOSIS

■ NOSOLOGY

Advances in biological and psychosocial understanding of substance use disorders (SUDs) have contributed to an evolution of SUD classification concurrent with the development of operational criteria and instruments such as DSM-IV (1) and the *Structured Clinical Interview for DSM-IV* (2). DSM-IV provides generic definitions of dependence, abuse, and withdrawal, as well as some specific definitions for substance-induced syndromes. A text revision of DSM-IV (DSM-IV-TR), published in 2000, especially elaborates on SUD categories that are difficult to diagnose.

■ DSM-IV CONTEXT

1. In DSM-IV, the term *substance* can refer to a drug of abuse, a medication, or a toxin, and it need not be limited to those that are psychoactive.
2. The term *organic* is absent from DSM-IV. The former *substance-induced organic mental disorders* are classified in the substance use disorders section. DSM-IV does distinguish substance-induced mental disorders from those that are due to a general medical condition and those that have no specified etiology.
3. DSM-IV diagnoses require the presence of "clinically significant distress and impairment in social, occupational, or other important areas of functioning."

4. DSM-IV diagnoses require that the condition is not due to a general medical condition and not better accounted for by another mental disorder.
5. DSM-IV-TR, the text revision of DSM-IV, does not alter the definitions of its mental disorders but instead provides updates to the accompanying descriptive text. The text notes that degrees of tolerance may vary by different central nervous system (CNS) functions. Tolerance does occur in phencyclidine (PCP) use, and DSM-IV-TR emphasizes the utility of lab tests, such as toxicology screens and gamma-glutamyltransferase assays, to detect relapse (see Chapter 6, Laboratory Findings and Diagnostic Instruments).

■ GENERIC DEFINITIONS AND DIAGNOSIS

Substance Dependence

Dependence is a collection of cognitive, behavioral, and physiological features that together signify continued use despite significant substance-related problems. It is a pattern of repeated self-administration that can result in tolerance, withdrawal, and compulsive drug-taking behavior. According to DSM-IV, the patient must, over a 12-month period, exhibit three behaviors from a seven-item polythetic criteria set (Table 4–1). Neither tolerance nor withdrawal is necessary or sufficient for a diagnosis of substance dependence. However, a past history of tolerance or withdrawal usually is associated with a more severe clinical course. Tolerance (the need for greatly increased amounts of a substance to produce a desired effect, or a greatly diminished effect with constant use of the same amount of the substance) may be difficult to discern from the patient's history when the substance used is of unknown purity. In such situations, quantitative laboratory tests may help. Withdrawal occurs when blood or tissue concentrations of a substance decline in an individual who had maintained pro-

---

TABLE 4–1.   **DSM-IV-TR criteria for substance dependence**

A maladaptive pattern of substance use, leading to clinically significant impairment or distress, as manifested by three (or more) of the following, occurring at any time in the same 12-month period:

(1) tolerance, as defined by either of the following:
   (a) a need for markedly increased amounts of the substance to achieve intoxication or desired effect
   (b) markedly diminished effect with continued use of the same amount of the substance
(2) withdrawal, as manifested by either of the following:
   (a) the characteristic withdrawal syndrome for the substance (refer to Criteria A and B of the criteria sets for withdrawal from the specific substances)
   (b) the same (or a closely related) substance is taken to relieve or avoid withdrawal symptoms
(3) the substance is often taken in larger amounts or over a longer period than was intended
(4) there is a persistent desire or unsuccessful efforts to cut down or control substance use
(5) a great deal of time is spent in activities necessary to obtain the substance (e.g., visiting multiple doctors or driving long distances), use the substance (e.g., chain-smoking), or recover from its effects
(6) important social, occupational, or recreational activities are given up or reduced because of substance use
(7) the substance use is continued despite knowledge of having a persistent or recurrent physical or psychological problem that is likely to have been caused or exacerbated by the substance (e.g., current cocaine use despite recognition of cocaine-induced depression, or continued drinking despite recognition that an ulcer was made worse by alcohol consumption)

Source.   Reprinted from American Psychiatric Association: *Diagnostic and Statistical Manual of Mental Disorders*, Fourth Edition, Text Revision. Washington, DC, American Psychiatric Association, 2000. Used with permission. Copyright 2000 American Psychiatric Association.

---

longed heavy use of the substance. In this state, the person will likely take the substance to relieve or to avoid unpleasant withdrawal symptoms.

According to DSM-IV, dependence can be noted as mild, moderate, or severe and remission may be noted to be partial, early partial, early full, sustained full, sustained partial, or full. The presence or absence of tolerance or withdrawal, other signs of physiological dependence, current use of agonist therapy, and placement in a controlled environment may be specified.

Substance Abuse

In DSM-IV, substance abuse includes continued use despite significant problems caused by the use in those who do not meet criteria for substance dependence. "Failure to fulfill major role obligations" is a criterion. To fulfill a criterion, the substance-related problem must have occurred repeatedly or persistently during the same 12-month period. The criteria for abuse do not include tolerance, withdrawal, or compulsive use (Table 4–2). Substance abuse cannot be applied to use of caffeine and nicotine. The term *abuse* should not be used as a blanket term for *use, misuse,* or *hazardous use.*

■ SUBSTANCE-INDUCED DISORDERS

Substance Intoxication

Substance intoxication (Table 4–3) is a reversible syndrome caused by recent exposure to a substance. It is often associated, and may be concurrently diagnosed, with substance abuse or dependence. The category does not apply to nicotine. Different substances (sometimes even different substance classes) may produce identical symptoms during intoxication.

Substance Withdrawal

Withdrawal (Table 4–4) is a behavioral, physiological, and cognitive state caused by the cessation of, or reduction in, heavy and prolonged substance use. Perhaps all withdrawing individuals crave the substance to reduce withdrawal symptoms. Signs and symp-

TABLE 4–2. **DSM-IV-TR criteria for substance abuse**

A. A maladaptive pattern of substance use leading to clinically significant impairment or distress, as manifested by one (or more) of the following, occurring within a 12-month period:
  (1) recurrent substance use resulting in a failure to fulfill major role obligations at work, school, or home (e.g., repeated absences or poor work performance related to substance use; substance-related absences, suspensions, or expulsions from school; neglect of children or household)
  (2) recurrent substance use in situations in which it is physically hazardous (e.g., driving an automobile or operating a machine when impaired by substance use)
  (3) recurrent substance-related legal problems (e.g., arrests for substance-related disorderly conduct)
  (4) continued substance use despite having persistent or recurrent social or interpersonal problems caused or exacerbated by the effects of the substance (e.g., arguments with spouse about consequences of intoxication, physical fights)
B. The symptoms have never met the criteria for substance dependence for this class of substance.

Source. Reprinted from American Psychiatric Association: *Diagnostic and Statistical Manual of Mental Disorders*, Fourth Edition, Text Revision. Washington, DC, American Psychiatric Association, 2000. Used with permission. Copyright 2000 American Psychiatric Association.

TABLE 4–3. **DSM-IV-TR criteria for substance intoxication**

A. The development of a reversible substance-specific syndrome due to recent ingestion of (or exposure to) a substance. **Note:** Different substances may produce similar or identical syndromes.
B. Clinically significant maladaptive behavioral or psychological changes that are due to the effect of the substance on the CNS (e.g., belligerence, mood lability, cognitive impairment, impaired judgment, impaired social or occupational functioning) and develop during or shortly after use of the substance.
C. The symptoms are not due to a general medical condition and are not better accounted for by another mental disorder.

Source. Reprinted from American Psychiatric Association: *Diagnostic and Statistical Manual of Mental Disorders*, Fourth Edition, Text Revision. Washington, DC, American Psychiatric Association, 2000. Used with permission. Copyright 2000 American Psychiatric Association.

TABLE 4–4. **DSM-IV-TR criteria for substance withdrawal**

A. The development of a substance-specific syndrome due to the cessation of (or reduction in) substance use that has been heavy and prolonged.
B. The substance-specific syndrome causes clinically significant distress or impairment in social, occupational, or other important areas of functioning.
C. The symptoms are not due to a general medical condition and are not better accounted for by another mental disorder.

Source. Reprinted from American Psychiatric Association: *Diagnostic and Statistical Manual of Mental Disorders*, Fourth Edition, Text Revision. Washington, DC, American Psychiatric Association, 2000. Used with permission. Copyright 2000 American Psychiatric Association.

toms vary according to the substance used; most symptoms are the opposite of those observed in intoxication by the same substance. Withdrawal is usually associated with substance dependence.

Substance-Induced Mental Disorders

Diagnosis of a substance-induced mental disorder requires evidence of intoxication or withdrawal. Some disorders can persist after the substance has been eliminated from the body, but symptoms lasting more than 4 weeks after acute intoxication or withdrawal are considered manifestations either of a primary mental disorder or a substance-induced persisting disorder. This differential diagnosis is complicated: withdrawal from some substances (e.g., sedatives) may partially mimic intoxication with others (e.g., amphetamines). The clinical import of a syndrome (e.g., depression with suicidal ideation) that is caused by a substance (e.g., cocaine) is in no way diminished. In most cases intoxication or withdrawal is distinguished from the substance-induced disorders of the same class because the symptoms in these latter disorders are in excess of those usually associated with intoxication or withdrawal from the substance and are severe enough to warrant independent clinical attention.

■ ALCOHOL

Alcohol Use Disorders

Although some groups have referred to alcohol dependence as *alcoholism*, the term has had no operational definition. It is important to distinguish abuse from dependence because although the abuser has some chance of drinking in a controlled manner, the dependent must become abstinent. Of course it is difficult to predict which abusers will become dependent: abstinence is safer and prevents progression to dependence.

Alcohol Dependence

The DSM-IV diagnostic criteria for alcohol dependence follow those for other substance disorders as delineated in Table 4–1. Specifying the presence of physiological dependence has prognostic value because it indicates a more severe clinical course (3), perhaps more so for alcohol withdrawal than for tolerance.

Alcohol Abuse

Fewer symptoms are required for a diagnosis of alcohol abuse than for dependence, and alcohol abuse is diagnosed only after dependence has been ruled out. Drinking when driving and a physician drinking before seeing patients are two examples of use of alcohol when a person is expected to fulfill role obligations. The development of medical and psychiatric complications related to alcohol use aid in diagnosis.

Alcohol-Induced Disorders

Alcohol Intoxication

Alcohol intoxication is time limited and reversible, and onset depends on tolerance, amount ingested, and amount absorbed. It is affected by interactions with other substances, medical status, and individual variation. Table 4–5 lists blood alcohol levels (BALs) and corresponding clinical features of a nonhabituated patient. For the habituated patient, chronic alcoholic presentation can vary greatly. Intoxication stages range from mild inebriation to anesthesia, coma, respiratory depression, and death. Relative to degree of tolerance, increasing BALs can lead to euphoria, mild coordination problems, ataxia, confusion, and decreased consciousness; BALs greater than 0.4 mg % can lead to anesthesia, coma, and death. Yet chronic heavy drinkers maintain high BALs with fewer effects. Alcohol intoxication may affect heart rate and electroencephalogram (EEG) readings and may cause nystagmus, slow reaction times, and behavioral changes including mood lability, impaired judgment, impaired social or occupational functioning, cognitive problems, and disinhibition of sexual or aggressive impulses. Intoxication with alcohol closely resembles sedative, hypnotic, or anxiolytic intoxication. Individual and cultural variations of tolerance may influence symptom presentation. Other neurological conditions such as cerebellar ataxia from multiple sclerosis may mimic some of the physiological signs and symptoms of alcohol intoxication. Alcohol idiosyncratic intoxication is not present in DSM-IV but could be diagnosed as an alcohol use disorder not otherwise specified (NOS). It should be noted that the odor of alcohol should not result in discounting the possibility that more than one substance is being used.

BAL (mg/dL)	Clinical presentation
30	Attention difficulties (mild), euphoria
50	Coordination problems, driving is legally impaired
100	Ataxia, drunk driving
200	Confusion, decreased consciousness
>400	Anesthesia, coma, death

TABLE 4–5. **Blood alcohol level (BAL) and typical clinical presentation in the nontolerant, alcohol-intoxicated patient**

Alcohol Withdrawal

Any relative drop in the BAL can precipitate withdrawal even during continuous alcohol consumption. Features include coarse tremor of hands, tongue, or eyelids; nausea or vomiting; malaise or weakness; autonomic hyperactivity; orthostatic hypotension; anxiety; depressed mood; irritability; transient hallucinations (generally poorly formed) or illusions; headache; and insomnia. The generalized tremor, which is coarse and of fast frequency (5–7 Hz), can worsen with motor activity or emotional stress; it is most likely to be observed on extension of the hands or tongue. Often patients complain of feeling shaky only inside. Careful attention should be paid to vital signs in a suspected alcoholic. Symptoms peak 24–48 hours after the last drink and subside in 5–7 days even without treatment. Insomnia and irritability may last 10 days or longer. The withdrawal symptoms may precipitate a relapse. Complications of major motor seizures ("rum fits") occur and are more likely to develop in those with a history of epilepsy and in those with other medical illnesses, malnutrition, fatigue, and depression.

Alcohol Intoxication or Withdrawal Delirium

Delirium tremens (d.t.'s) can result from alcohol withdrawal or intoxication. It differs from uncomplicated withdrawal in that it includes a delirium that may involve abnormal perceptions, agitation, terror, insomnia, mild fever, or autonomic instability. Hallucinations may be auditory and of a persecutory nature, or they may be kinesthetic, such as tactile sensations of crawling insects. Yet a wide variation of presentations can occur, from quiet confusion, agitation, and peculiar behavior lasting several weeks to marked abnormal behavior, vivid terrifying delusions, and other disorders of perception. The d.t.'s can appear suddenly but usually manifests gradually 2–3 days after cessation of drinking, with peak intensity on day 4 or 5. It is usually benign and short-lived: the majority of cases subside after 3 days; subacute symptoms may last 4–5 weeks. Although early reports stated that up to 20% of cases may end fatally, later reports show a fatality rate that may be less than

1%. The d.t.'s is associated with infections, subdural hematomas, trauma, liver disease, and metabolic disorders, and the cause of death is usually infectious fat emboli or cardiac arrhythmias (usually associated with hyperkalemia, hyperpyrexia, and poor hydration). The d.t.'s generally occurs in withdrawing alcoholics who have been heavy drinkers for 5–15 years.

Alcohol Withdrawal Seizures

Alcohol lowers seizure threshold. Alcohol withdrawal seizures that are not a part of d.t.'s generally occur 7–38 hours after the last alcohol use in chronic drinkers, mostly about 24 hours after. Half of these occur in bursts of two to six grand mal seizures. Fewer than 3% of patients in withdrawal develop status epilepticus. A total of 10% of all chronic drinkers endure a grand mal seizure; one-third of all who seize progress to d.t.'s, and one-fiftieth of all who seize progress to status epilepticus (4). Focal seizures suggest a focal lesion, which may indicate trauma or epilepsy. Hypomagnesemia, respiratory alkalosis, hypoglycemia, and increased intracellular sodium levels have been associated with these seizures. Serum magnesium levels should be tested in alcoholic patients who develop seizures. Any seizures predict a complicated withdrawal period.

Alcohol-Persisting Dementia

Prolonged and heavy use of alcohol may be followed by dementia. Diagnosis is confirmed by its presence at least 3 weeks after ending alcohol intake. In this condition, unlike alcohol amnestic disorder, cognitive impairment affects more than memory function, and no cause other than alcohol is found.

Alcohol-Induced Persisting Amnestic Disorder
(Korsakoff's Syndrome)

Thiamine (vitamin B_1) deficiency associated with prolonged heavy use of alcohol produces alcohol-induced persisting amnestic disorder (Korsakoff's syndrome) and its associated neurological deficits (peripheral neuropathy, cerebellar ataxia, and myopathy). It often follows acute Wernicke's encephalopathy (confusion, ataxia, nystagmus, ophthalmoplegia, and other neurological signs). As Wernicke's encephalopathy subsides, severe impairment of anterograde and retrograde memory remains; confabulation is common. Early treatment of Wernicke's encephalopathy with large doses of thiamine may prevent Korsakoff's syndrome. Unlike other dementias, in this syndrome intellectual function is preserved.

Alcohol-Induced Psychotic Disorder With
Delusions or Hallucinations

Alcohol-induced psychotic disorder with hallucinations is far more common than with delusions. The hallucinosis consists of vivid and persistent hallucinations, usually within 48 hours after reduction of alcohol in dependent patients. Auditory or visual hallucinations can occur. This disorder may last several weeks or months. Hallucinations may range from sounds (e.g., clicks, roaring, humming, ringing bells, chanting) to threatening or derogatory voices. One derogatory remark may develop into relentlessly persisting auditory accusations and commands by several voices. Patients usually respond with fear, anxiety, and agitation. Diagnosis is usually based on a history of heavy alcohol use, lack of formal thought disorder, and lack of psychosis in the personal or family history. In the majority of cases, the symptoms recede in a few hours to days, the patients fully realizing the perceptions were imaginary. Rarely, patients develop a quiet, chronic, paranoid delusional state indistinguishable from frank schizophrenia from which remission would not be expected after 6 months. Overall, differential diagnosis includes d.t.'s, withdrawal syndrome, paranoid psychosis, and borderline transient psychotic episodes. In contrast to d.t.'s, these hallucinations usually occur in a clear consciousness. Lack of autonomic symptoms differentiates the syndrome from withdrawal.

Alcohol-Induced Sexual Dysfunction

Alcohol broadly affects reproductive function, generally in proportion to the magnitude of use. Contrary to myth, both men and women have decreased sexual function when they are alcohol dependent.

Blackouts

Blackouts are periods of amnesia during periods of intoxication (by most CNS depressants) despite a state of consciousness that seems normal. They may occur in nonalcoholics during heavy drinking or at any time during alcohol dependence. Severity and duration of use correlate with blackout occurrence.

■ SEDATIVES, HYPNOTICS, AND ANXIOLYTICS

Sedative, hypnotic, and anxiolytic substances include benzodiazepines, carbamates (e.g., glutethimide, meprobamate), barbiturates (e.g., secobarbital), and barbiturate-like hypnotics (e.g., glutethimide, methaqualone). This class includes all prescription sleeping medications (e.g., chloral hydrate, paraldehyde) and almost all prescription anxiolytics. The nonbenzodiazepine anxiolytics (e.g., buspirone, gepirone) are not included. Polysubstance abusers frequently self-medicate with sedatives to treat undesirable effects of cocaine or amphetamines. Definitions for this class and other classes of drugs follow the generic definitions of dependence and abuse presented in Tables 4–1 and 4–2. This class of substances produces secondary clinical syndromes that generally parallel those secondary to alcohol, but their pharmacokinetics differ from alcohol in important ways. It is important to distinguish legitimate use of these medications from adaptation and maladaptive habituation and from illegal use.

Sedative, Hypnotic, or Anxiolytic Dependence

A diagnosis of dependence on sedatives, hypnotics, or anxiolytics should be considered only when, in addition to having physiological dependence, the individual using the substance shows evidence of a range of problems (e.g., an individual who has developed drug-seeking behavior to the extent that important activities are given up or reduced to obtain the substance). In this class of drugs, degree of physical dependence is closely related to dosage and length of use. For example, an individual who has taken benzodiazepines for long periods of time at prescribed and therapeutic doses and abruptly discontinues use may show signs of tolerance and withdrawal in the absence of a diagnosis of substance dependence.

Sedative, Hypnotic, or Anxiolytic Intoxication

Memory impairment, which can be quite disturbing to the individual, is a prominent feature of sedative, hypnotic, or anxiolytic intoxication and is most often characterized by an anterograde amnesia that resembles alcoholic blackouts. As with other CNS depressants, one (or more) of the following signs develop during, or shortly after, sedative, hypnotic, or anxiolytic use: slurred speech, incoordination, unsteady gait, nystagmus, impairment in attention or memory, or stupor or coma.

Sedative, Hypnotic, or Anxiolytic Withdrawal

Sedative, hypnotic, or anxiolytic withdrawal is a characteristic syndrome that develops after a decrease in intake after regular use. Even a low dose of diazepam (5 to 10 mg) over time can result in significant withdrawal on abrupt cessation. Benzodiazepine abuse can involve several hundred milligrams of diazepam or its equivalent. Individuals who tolerate such dosages are dependent and require active substance abuse treatment with medications. As with alcohol, benzodiazepine withdrawal includes two or more symptoms such as autonomic hyperactivity, tremor, insomnia, anxiety, nausea, vomiting, and psychomotor agitation. Relief on administration of any sedative-hypnotic agent supports a diagnosis of withdrawal. Grand mal seizures occur in 20%–30% of untreated individuals. The withdrawal syndrome produced by substances in this class may present as a life-threatening delirium. In severe withdrawal, perceptual disturbances can occur (if the person's reality testing is intact and sensorium clear, the specifier "with perceptual disturbances" should be noted). The timing and severity of the syndrome depends on the pharmacokinetics and pharmacodynamics of the substance. For drugs with longer half-lives, symptoms may develop more slowly than for those with shorter half-lives. There may be additional longer-term symptoms at a much lower level of intensity that persist for several months. As with alcohol, lingering withdrawal symptoms (e.g., anxiety, moodiness, and trouble sleeping) can be mistaken for non–substance-induced anxiety or depressive disorders (e.g., generalized anxiety disorder).

Sedative, Hypnotic, or Anxiolytic Withdrawal Delirium

Sedative, hypnotic, or anxiolytic withdrawal delirium is characterized by disturbances in consciousness and cognition from visual, tactile, or auditory hallucinations. When present, withdrawal delirium should be the diagnosis rather than withdrawal.

■ OPIOIDS

Opioid Dependence

Most individuals with opioid dependence have significant tolerance and experience withdrawal on abrupt discontinuation. The diagnosis requires the presence of features that reflect compulsive use without legitimate medical purpose or use of doses that are greatly in excess of that needed for pain relief.

Opioid Abuse

Dependence, rather than abuse, should be considered when problems related to opioid use are accompanied by evidence of tolerance, withdrawal, or compulsive behavior related to the use of opioids.

Opioid-Induced Disorders

Opioids are less likely than most other drugs of abuse to produce psychiatric symptoms and may reduce such symptoms. Opioid intoxication and opioid withdrawal are distinguished from the other opioid-induced disorders because the symptoms in these latter disorders are in excess of those usually associated with intoxication or withdrawal and are severe enough to warrant independent clinical attention.

Opioid-Induced Intoxication

The magnitude of the behavioral and physiological changes that result from opioid use depends on the dose and on the characteristics of the user. Symptoms of intoxication usually last as long as the half-life of the drug. Intoxication is marked by miosis or, if severe, by mydriasis (due to anoxia). Drowsiness, slurred speech, and impairment in attention and memory are other signs. Aggression and violence are rarely seen. When hallucinations occur in the absence of intact reality testing, a diagnosis of opioid-induced psychotic disorder with hallucinations should be considered. Intoxication by alcohol, sedatives, hypnotics, or anxiolytics resembles opioid intoxication, but it does not produce miosis or a response to a naloxone challenge.

Opioid overdose is an emergent situation that can be quickly diagnosed. It presents as coma, shock, pinpoint pupils (dilation in severe cases), and depressed respiration that may lead to death. It rapidly responds to Narcan (naloxone), an opioid receptor antagonist; a lack of response to naloxone undermines a presumed diagnosis of opioid overdose. However, if other classes of drugs are producing the altered mental state, naloxone will produce only a partial improvement. Opioid intoxication is distinguished from alcohol and sedative intoxication by presence of pupillary constriction and positive toxicological test results.

Opioid Withdrawal

Opioid withdrawal is a syndrome that follows a relative reduction in heavy and prolonged use. The syndrome begins within 6–8 hours after the last dose and peaks at 48–72 hours, and symptoms disappear in 7–10 days. Opioid withdrawal includes signs and symptoms that are opposite the acute agonist effects: lacrimation, rhinorrhea, pupillary dilation, piloerection, diaphoresis, diarrhea, yawning, mild hypertension, tachycardia, fever, and insomnia. A flulike syndrome includes complaints, demands, and drug seeking. Although intense, uncomplicated withdrawal is usually not life threatening unless there is a severe underlying disorder such as cardiac disease. The anxiety and restlessness associated with opioid withdrawal resemble symptoms seen in sedative, hypnotic, or anxiolytic withdrawal. However, opioid withdrawal is also accompanied by rhinorrhea, lacrimation, and mydriasis, which are not seen in sedative-type withdrawal (see Table 4–6 for the full criteria set).

■ COCAINE

Cocaine can be administered using coca leaves (chewed), coca paste (smoked), cocaine hydrochloride powder (inhaled or injected), and cocaine alkaloid, freebase or crack (smoked). Speedballing (mixing cocaine and heroin) is particularly dangerous due to potentiation of respiratory depressant effects. Cocaine-induced states should be distinguished from the symptoms of schizophrenia (paranoid type), bipolar and other mood disorders, generalized anxiety disorder, and panic disorder.

Cocaine Dependence

Exposure to cocaine can quickly produce dependence. An early sign is a growing difficulty resisting the drug. With its short half-life, frequent use is needed to keep a high. Complications of chronic use are common and include paranoia, aggression, anxiety, depression, and weight loss. Tolerance occurs with repeated use by any

TABLE 4–6.	DSM-IV-TR diagnostic criteria for opioid withdrawal

A. Either of the following:
  (1) cessation of (or reduction in) opioid use that has been heavy and prolonged (several weeks or longer)
  (2) administration of an opioid antagonist after a period of opioid use
B. Three (or more) of the following, developing within minutes to several days after Criterion A:
  (1) dysphoric mood
  (2) nausea or vomiting
  (3) muscle aches
  (4) lacrimation or rhinorrhea
  (5) pupillary dilation, piloerection, or sweating
  (6) diarrhea
  (7) yawning
  (8) fever
  (9) insomnia
C. The symptoms in Criterion B cause clinically significant distress or impairment in social, occupational, or other important areas of functioning.
D. The symptoms are not due to a general medical condition and are not better accounted for by another mental disorder.

Source. Reprinted from American Psychiatric Association: *Diagnostic and Statistical Manual of Mental Disorders*, Fourth Edition, Text Revision. Washington, DC, American Psychiatric Association, 2000. Used with permission. Copyright 2000 American Psychiatric Association.

route of administration. Withdrawal symptoms, particularly dysphoria, can be seen but are usually transitory and associated with high-dose use.

Cocaine Abuse

The intensity and frequency of cocaine use is less in cases of abuse than of dependence. Episodes of clinically significant use often occur around paydays or special occasions, leading to a pattern of brief periods (hours to days) of heavy use and longer periods (weeks to months) of nonsignificant use or abstinence. Dependence, rather than abuse, should be considered when tolerance, withdrawal, or compulsive behavior related to obtaining and using the drug accompany use.

Cocaine Intoxication

Cocaine intoxication is a state that develops during, or shortly after, cocaine use. After an initial high, cocaine intoxication produces one or more of the following effects: euphoria with enhanced vigor, gregariousness, hyperactivity, restlessness, hypervigilance, interpersonal sensitivity, talkativeness, anxiety, tension, alertness, grandiosity, stereotyped and repetitive behavior, anger, and impaired judgment, and in the case of chronic intoxication, affective blunting with fatigue or sadness and social withdrawal. These features occur with two or more of the following: tachycardia or bradycardia; pupillary dilation; elevated or lowered blood pressure; perspiration or chills; nausea or vomiting; evidence of weight loss; psychomotor agitation or retardation; muscular weakness, respiratory depression, chest pain, or cardiac arrhythmias; and confusion, seizures, dyskinesias, dystonias, or coma. Cocaine's stimulant effects such as euphoria, tachycardia, hypertension, and psychomotor activity are more commonly seen than its depressant effects (sadness, bradycardia, hypotension, and psychomotor retardation), which emerge only with chronic high-dose use. Binges are highly reinforcing and may lead to psychosis or death. Cocaine's effects on the noradrenergic system are significant and in the overdose setting are associated with muscular twitching, rhabdomyolysis, seizures, cerebrovascular accidents, myocardial infarctions, arrhythmias, and respiratory failure.

Intravenous or freebase use greatly intensifies the rush. The half-life of cocaine used intravenously is less than 90 minutes, with euphoric effects lasting 15–20 minutes. Most cocaine is hydrolyzed to benzoylecgonine, which may be detected in the urine for up to 36 hours. Metabolism is slowed when cocaine is combined with alcohol, in which case there is an 18- to 25-fold greater chance of death than from cocaine alone. Smoked freebase has an onset of intense euphoria within seconds because it passes directly from the lungs to the systemic circulation. Euphoric effects depend on concentration and on the slope of the peak concentration (5).

Tolerance to the euphoric effects develops during a binge; however, there is less tolerance for adverse experiences such as increasing anxiety, panic, or frank delirium. With prolonged cocaine administration, a transient delusional psychosis simulating paranoid schizophrenia can be seen. Usually the symptoms remit, although heavy prolonged use or predisposing psychopathology may lead to persisting psychosis. Generally higher dosages differentiate overdose from intoxication. Amphetamine or PCP intoxication can often be distinguished from cocaine intoxication only by toxicological studies.

Cocaine Withdrawal

Cocaine withdrawal is accompanied by dysphoric mood, irritability, anxiety, fatigue, insomnia or hyposomnia, vivid and unpleasant dreams, and psychomotor agitation. Anhedonia and drug craving may be present. Withdrawal occurs more than 24 hours after cessation of use and generally peaks in 2–4 days (yet irritability and depression may continue for months). Acute withdrawal symptoms are often seen after periods of repetitive high-dose use. These periods are characterized by intense and unpleasant feelings of lassitude and depression, perhaps with suicidal ideation, and generally require days of rest and recuperation. EEG abnormalities may be present.

Cocaine Delirium

Cocaine delirium may occur within 24 hours of use. It may produce tactile and olfactory hallucinations, although violent or aggressive behavior is more frequent. Cocaine delirium is self-limited and usually resolves after 6 hours.

Cocaine Delusional Disorder

Cocaine delusional disorder is marked by rapidly developing persecutory delusions that may be accompanied by body image distortion, misperception of people's faces, formication, and aggression or violence.

■ AMPHETAMINES

The class of amphetamines includes substances with a substituted-phenylethylamine structure (e.g., amphetamine, dextroamphetamine, and methamphetamine [speed]) and those that have amphetamine-like action but are structurally different (e.g., methylphenidate and most agents used as appetite suppressants). Signs and symptoms of amphetamine use parallel those of cocaine use, although effects may last longer than with cocaine. Amphetamine psychosis can resemble acute paranoid schizophrenia and frequently occurs with visual hallucinations. Patterns of use include the predominant oral administration in pill form and resemble cocaine use, with binge episodes alternating with crash symptoms. Peripheral sympathomimetic effects may be quite potent.

Amphetamine Intoxication

Amphetamine intoxication follows use of amphetamine or a related substance. Behavioral and psychological changes are accompanied by at least two of the following: tachycardia or bradycardia, mydriasis, hypertension or hypotension, perspiration or chills, nausea or vomiting, weight loss, psychomotor agitation or retardation, muscular weakness, respiratory depression, and chest pain. Confusion, arrhythmias, seizures, dyskinesias, dystonias, or coma may follow. The state begins no more than 1 hour after use, depending on the drug and method of delivery. Perceptual disturbances should be specified when hallucinations or illusions occur in the absence of a delirium and with intact reality testing. If such disturbances occur in the absence of reality testing, consider classifying them as amphetamine-induced psychotic disorder, with hallucinations.

Differential Diagnosis of
Amphetamine-Induced Disorders

Amphetamine-induced disorders may resemble primary mental disorders. A very difficult differential diagnosis is between amphetamine-induced psychosis and schizophrenia (6). Intoxication by cocaine, hallucinogens, and PCP may cause similar symptoms and can sometimes be distinguished from amphetamine intoxication only by urine or serum toxicology, although mydriasis, history of recent drug use, and speed of onset may provide clues. Dependence on or abuse of amphetamines should be distinguished from dependence on or abuse of cocaine, PCP, and hallucinogens.

■ PCP AND KETAMINE

Originally an anesthetic, PCP ("angel dust" or the "PeaCe" pill) has become a street drug with epidemic use in some urban areas. Variations include ketamine (ketalar) and the thiophene analogue of PCP (TCP). These substances can be used orally or intravenously and can be smoked and inhaled. PCP is often mixed with other substances such as amphetamines, cannabis, cocaine, or hallucinogens.

PCP Dependence

Dependence may have a rapid onset, and effects are generally unpredictable. DSM-IV diagnosis of PCP dependence includes the first seven items of the generic definition of substance dependence (see Table 4–1), but criteria 2a and 2b may not apply because a clear-cut withdrawal pattern is difficult to establish. As with hallucinogens, adverse reactions to PCP may be more common among individuals with preexisting mental disorders.

PCP Abuse

PCP abusers may fail to fulfill role obligations because of intoxication. They may use in situations where doing so is physically hazardous. Recurrent social or interpersonal problems may result because of intoxicated behavior or a chaotic lifestyle, legal problems, or arguments with significant others.

PCP-Induced Disorders

PCP Intoxication

Intoxication begins by 5 minutes after use and peaks in 30 minutes. PCP intoxication produces affective instability, stereotypies, bizarre aggression, altered perception, disorganization, and confusion. Signs include hypertension, numbness, muscular rigidity, ataxia, and, at high doses, hyperthermia and involuntary movements followed by amnesia, coma, and analgesia; seizures and respiratory depression occur at the highest doses (greater than 20 mg). Milder intoxication resolves after 8–20 hours, but because of the fat solubility of PCP, low-level intoxication may persist for many days. Mydriasis and nystagmus (vertical more than horizontal) are characteristic of PCP use and help confirm diagnosis. Perceptual disturbances should be specified if present.

PCP-Induced Psychosis

PCP-induced psychosis, the most common PCP-induced disorder, may occur in predisposed individuals. It may be indistinguishable from a psychotic episode. Chronic psychosis may occur along with long-term neuropsychological deficits.

Differential Diagnosis of PCP-Induced Disorders

PCP-induced disorders may resemble primary mental disorders. Recurring episodes of psychotic or mood symptoms due to PCP may mimic schizophrenia or mood disorders. PCP use establishes a role for the substance in producing a mentally disordered state but does not rule out the co-occurrence of other primary mental disorders. Although rapid onset of symptoms also suggests PCP use rather than a mental disorder, it may be that PCP use induces syndromes in individuals with preexisting disease. The course and the absence of a history of the disorder may aid this differentiation. Drug-related violence or impaired judgment may co-occur with, or may mimic aspects of, conduct disorder or antisocial personality disorder. Again, a history of disordered conduct may help to clarify the situation. PCP users often use other drugs, thus comorbid abuse of or dependence on other substances must be considered.

■ HALLUCINOGENS

Hallucinogens are a diverse group of substances that include indoleamine derivatives (lysergic acid diethylamide [LSD], morning glory seeds), phenylalkylamine derivatives (mescaline, 2,5-dimethoxy-4-methylamphetamine [STP], and ring-substituted amphetamines such as MDA [old ecstasy], MDMA [new ecstasy], and MDEA), indole alkaloids (psilocybin, dimethyltryptamine [DMT]), and miscellaneous other compounds. Excluded from this group are PCP, cannabis, and delta-9-tetrahydrocannabinol (THC). Hallucinogens are usually taken orally, although DMT is smoked, and use by injection does occur.

Hallucinogen Dependence

There are no specific criteria for hallucinogen dependence, and some of the generic dependence criteria do not apply, whereas others require explanation. Hallucinogen use is often limited to only a few times a week even among individuals meeting full criteria for dependence. Tolerance to the euphoric and psychedelic effects of hallucinogens develop rapidly but not to the autonomic effects (mydriasis, hyperreflexia, hypertension, increased body temperature, piloerection, and tachycardia). Cross-tolerance exists between LSD and other hallucinogens (e.g., psilocybin and mescaline). Withdrawal has not been demonstrated, but clear reports of craving after stopping hallucinogen use are known. Some MDMA users describe a hangover the day after use that includes insomnia, fatigue, drowsiness, sore jaw muscles from teeth clenching, loss of balance, and headaches. Some of the reported adverse effects may be due to adulterant or substitute substances such as strychnine, PCP, or amphetamine.

Hallucinogen Intoxication

In the state of hallucinogen intoxication, perceptual changes occur alongside full alertness during or shortly after hallucinogen use. Changes include subjective intensification of perceptions, depersonalization, derealization, illusions, hallucinations, and synesthesias. DSM-IV criteria require the presence of two of the given physiological signs. At low doses, the perceptual changes often do not include hallucinations. Synesthesias (a blending of senses) may result in, for example, sounds being seen. Hallucinations are usually visual: often of geometric forms, and sometimes of persons and objects. Auditory or tactile hallucinations are rare. Reality testing is usually preserved. Intoxication should be differentiated from amphetamine or PCP intoxication, which can be accomplished through toxicological tests. Intoxication with anticholinergics (e.g., trihexyphenidyl [Artane]) can produce hallucinations, but they are often associated with fever, dry mouth and skin, flushed face, and visual disturbances.

Hallucinogen Psychotic Disorder

Hallucinogen psychotic disorder may be brief or lead to a long-lasting psychotic episode that is difficult to distinguish from schizophreniform disorder.

Posthallucinogen Perception Disorder

Posthallucinogen perception disorder (flashbacks) following cessation of hallucinogen use is the reexperiencing of one or more of the same perceptual symptoms experienced while originally intoxicated. It usually is fleeting but rarely may be more lasting and persistent. It may be marked by noticing trails, intensified flashes of colors, auditory visual hallucinations, and false perceptions of movement. Symptoms may be triggered by stress, drug use (including drugs such as cannabis), emergence into a dark environment, or even by intention. If the person's interpretation of the etiology of the state is delusional, the diagnosis is psychotic disorder not otherwise specified. Hallucinogen intoxication is distinguished from this disorder by temporal relation to use. Also, in posthallucinogen perception disorder, the individual does not believe that the perception represents external reality, whereas a person with a psychotic disorder often believes that the perception is real. Hallucinogen persisting perception disorder may be distinguished from migraine, epilepsy, or a neurological condition by taking the individual's neuro-ophthalmological history, a physical examination, and using appropriate laboratory evaluation.

■ CANNABIS

In the cannabis class, the substances most commonly used include marijuana, hashish, and purified delta-9-tetrahydrocannabinol (THC). Usually smoked, these substances may also be mixed with food and eaten.

Cannabis Dependence

Dependence is marked by daily, or almost daily, compulsive cannabis use. Tolerance to most of the effects of cannabis has been reported in chronic users, but these patients do not generally develop physiological dependence, and physiological dependence is not a criterion for diagnosis in DSM-IV. Withdrawal after heavy use is not clinically significant.

Cannabis Abuse

Abuse is characterized by episodic use with maladaptive behavior. When significant levels of tolerance are present, or when psychological or physical problems are associated with cannabis in the context of compulsive use, dependence should be considered rather than abuse.

Cannabis-Induced Disorders

Cannabis Intoxication

Cannabis intoxication includes effects of the drug that are determined in major ways by the interaction of drug, person, and setting (route of administration, pharmacodynamics, and pharmacokinetics). Intoxication after smoking cannabis peaks after 10–30 minutes and lasts about 3 hours; metabolites may have a half-life of approximately 50 hours. Because most cannabinoids are fat soluble, their effects may occasionally persist or reoccur for 12–24 hours as a result of a slow release from fatty tissue or to enterohepatic circulation. Intoxication includes euphoria, anxiety, suspiciousness or paranoid ideation, sensation of slowed time, impaired judgment, and social withdrawal. Inappropriate laughter, panic attacks, and dysphoric affect may occur. Adverse reactions may be more common in those with psychiatric disorders or those frightened about the drug-taking situation. At least two of the following signs develop within 2 hours of use: 1) conjunctival injection, 2) increased appetite, 3) dry mouth, and 4) tachycardia. For differentiation, note that intoxication by alcohol or a sedative, hypnotic, or anxiolytic substance usually decreases appetite, increases aggressive behavior, and produces nystagmus or ataxia. In low doses, hallucinogens may result in symptoms that resemble cannabis intoxication. PCP intoxication is much more likely to cause ataxia and aggressive behavior. DSM-IV provides a specifier for intoxication with perceptual disturbances; although if hallucinations occur without intact reality testing, substance-induced psychotic disorder, with hallucinations, should be the diagnosis.

Cannabis Delusional Disorder

Cannabis delusional disorder is a syndrome (usually with persecutory delusions) that develops shortly after cannabis use. It may be associated with marked anxiety, depersonalization, and emotional lability and may be misdiagnosed as schizophrenia. Subsequent amnesia for the episode can occur.

Cannabis-Induced Mental Disorders

Cannabis-induced mental disorders are diverse. Chronic use can resemble dysthymic disorder. Acute adverse reactions to cannabis should be differentiated from panic, major depressive disorder, delusional disorder, bipolar disorder, and paranoid schizophrenia.

■ NICOTINE

Nicotine has euphoric effects and reinforcement properties similar to those of cocaine and opioids. Its effects can follow use of all forms of tobacco and prescription medications containing nicotine (nicotine gum and patch).

Nicotine Dependence

For nicotine, some of the generic dependence criteria do not appear to apply, and other criteria need explanation. Tolerance is the absence of nausea, dizziness, and other characteristic symptoms despite the use of substantial amounts of nicotine, or it is a diminished effect observed with continued use of the same amount. In making the diagnosis, it should be recalled that spending a great deal of time attempting to procure nicotine is likely rare. An example of giving up important social, occupational, or recreational activities is the avoidance of an activity because it occurs in smoking-restricted areas.

Nicotine-Induced Disorders

Nicotine Withdrawal

Nicotine withdrawal develops after the abrupt cessation of, or reduction in, the use of nicotine following a prolonged period (at least several weeks) of daily use. The withdrawal syndrome includes four or more of the following effects: dysphoric or depressed mood; insomnia; irritability, frustration, or anger; anxiety; difficulty concentrating; restlessness or impatience; decreased heart rate; and increased appetite or weight gain. Heart rate decreases by 5–12 beats per minute in the first few days after cessation, and weight increases an average of 2–3 kg in the year after cessation. Mild withdrawal may occur after switching to low-tar low-nicotine cigarettes or after stopping the use of chewing tobacco, nicotine gum, or patches.

Differential Diagnosis of Nicotine-Induced Mental Disorders

The symptoms of nicotine withdrawal overlap with those of other withdrawal syndromes; caffeine intoxication; anxiety, mood, and sleep disorders; and medication-induced akathisia. Reduction of symptoms associated with the replacement of nicotine confirms the diagnosis.

■ INHALANTS

The class of inhaled substances includes the aliphatic and aromatic hydrocarbons found in substances such as gasoline, glue, paint thinners, and spray paints. Less commonly used are halogenated hydrocarbons (in cleaners, correction fluid, spray-can propellants) and other volatile compounds containing esters, ketones, and glycols. It is usually difficult to determine the exact substance responsible for the disorder. Diagnosis is always confirmed by toxicology. Although there may be subtle differences in the effects of the compounds, not enough is known about their effects to distinguish among them. Indeed these drugs may be used interchangeably, and use may depend on availability and experience. Nonetheless, all are capable of producing dependence, abuse, and intoxication. There are no specific criteria sets for dependence or abuse of inhalants; this is partially the result of the uncertain existence of tolerance or withdrawal syndromes. A possible withdrawal syndrome beginning 24–48 hours after cessation of use and lasting from 2 to 5 days has been described, with symptoms including sleep disturbances, tremor, irritability, diaphoresis, nausea, and fleeting illusions.

Inhalant-Induced Disorders

Inhalant intoxication is clinically significant maladaptive behavioral or psychological changes (e.g., belligerence, assaultiveness, apathy, impaired judgment, impaired social or occupational functioning) that develop during or shortly after exposure. The maladaptive changes are accompanied by signs that include dizziness or visual disturbances (blurred vision or diplopia), nystagmus, incoordination, slurred speech, unsteady gait, tremor, and euphoria. Higher doses of inhalants may lead to the development of lethargy and psychomotor retardation, generalized muscle weakness, depressed reflexes, stupor, or coma.

Differential Diagnosis of Inhalant-Induced Disorders

Inhalant-induced disorders may be characterized by symptoms that resemble primary mental disorders. Mild to moderate intoxication can be similar to intoxication by alcohol, sedatives, hypnotics, or anxiolytics. Chronic users are likely to use other substances frequently and heavily, further complicating the diagnosis. History of the drug used and characteristic findings (including odor of solvent or paint residue) may differentiate inhalant intoxication from other substance intoxications. Rapid onset and resolution may also differentiate inhalant intoxication from other mental disorders and neurological conditions. Industrial workers may occasionally be accidentally exposed to volatile chemicals and suffer physiological intoxication. For such toxin exposures, the appropriate category is other substance–related disorders.

■ CAFFEINE

Caffeine is widely used in the form of coffee, tea, cola, chocolate, and cocoa, and also in over-the-counter analgesics, cold preparations, and stimulants. There is no DSM-IV diagnosis for caffeine dependence or abuse. Withdrawal headaches may occur, but they are usually not severe enough to require treatment. Intoxication can lead to restlessness, nervousness, excitement, insomnia, flushing, diuresis, and gastrointestinal complaints. Doses leading to intoxication can vary. At high doses, there can be psychosis, arrhythmias, and psychomotor agitation. Mild sensory disturbances can occur at higher doses; at enormous doses, grand mal seizures and respiratory failure may occur. Intoxication may not occur despite high caffeine intake because of tolerance. DSM-IV criteria recognize other caffeine-induced disorders including anxiety disorder and sleep disorder, and there is also a category for caffeine-related disorder not otherwise specified.

Differential Diagnosis of Caffeine-Induced Disorders

The bulk of disorders that can be differentiated from caffeine-induced mental disorders include medical conditions that mimic caffeine intoxication. The temporal relationship of the symptoms to increased caffeine use or to abstinence from caffeine helps to establish the diagnosis. The following can cause a clinical picture that is similar to that of caffeine intoxication: manic episodes; panic disorder; generalized anxiety disorder; amphetamine intoxication; sedative, hypnotic, or anxiolytic withdrawal or nicotine withdrawal; sleep disorders; and medication-induced side effects (e.g., akathisia).

■ OTHER (OR UNKNOWN) SUBSTANCE–RELATED DISORDERS

DSM-IV includes categories for dependence, abuse, intoxication, withdrawal, delirium, psychosis with delusions, psychosis with hallucinations, persisting dementia or amnesia, disordered mood, anxiety, sexual dysfunction, and disordered sleep that result from use of a small number of substances. Such include amyl nitrate, anticholinergics, gamma-hydroxybutyrate (GHB), corticosteroids, anabolic steroids, antihistamines, antiparkinsonian agents, and substances that are unknown at the time of presentation.

GHB is a CNS depressant that is used in some countries (but not the United States) as an anesthetic. It is increasingly used worldwide as a recreational drug by party and nightclub attendees and bodybuilders, and it also may be used as a date rape drug. It has been marketed to bodybuilders as a growth hormone releaser. Known as "Liquid Ecstasy," and "Cherry Menth," GHB increases CNS dopamine levels and has effects on the endogenous opioid system. GHB toxicity includes coma, seizures, respiratory depression, vomiting, anesthesia, and amnesia (7). Full recovery is usually the case, but the toxic state is critical.

■ POLYSUBSTANCE DEPENDENCE

Polysubstance dependence is the DSM-IV category that is used when an individual has repeatedly used substances from at least three classes (with the exception of nicotine and caffeine) within the last year without one predominating. Dependence is global and not on any one drug. Patients often downplay use of secondary drugs. For example, without a thorough substance use history, a diagnosed cocaine abuser may develop alcohol withdrawal unexpectedly.

■ DRUG COMBINATIONS

Often one drug is used to counterbalance the side effects or to potentiate the effect of another drug. Speedballing, the intravenous combination of heroin and cocaine, is often lethal but is known to mute cocaine dysphoria. Glutethimide (Doriden) and cocaine are often combined, potentiating respiratory depression. Pentazocine (Talwin) and diphenhydramine (Benadryl) (the "T's and Blues") are prescription medications that produce intoxication when combined. Virtually any combination of alcohol and other drugs is seen. Marijuana use is often so pervasive among polysubstance abusers that it is not perceived as a drug of abuse.

■ MAKING A DIAGNOSIS

Diagnostic Dilemmas

The substance-abusing patient presents with medical, neurological, and psychiatric disturbances that need careful systematic assessment. This difficulty with differential diagnoses should instill some degree of humility and conservatism. Conservative management with a careful review of medical, psychiatric, and substance abuse histories; physical and mental status examinations; laboratory tests; and third-party information can often clarify the diagnoses. In other cases, only time and observation clarify the etiology.

Signs and Symptoms

The care of substance-abusing patients and the diagnosis of their conditions require attention to physical signs and symptoms. At the outset, when differentiating among overdose, withdrawal, chronic organicity, and psychiatric diagnoses, one should rule out or treat life-threatening conditions first. For example, tachycardia and fever may indicate infection, withdrawal, or drug toxicity. An abnormal pulse may indicate intoxication with sympathomimetic drugs, withdrawal from CNS depressants, or arrhythmia from overdose. Bradycardia could indicate opioid intoxication, severe head trauma, or cardiac conduction delays. Abnormal pupil size or occulogyric movements can help clarify various drug overdose situations. Pinpoint pupils in a comatose patient may signal opioid overdose. Mydriasis is associated with sympathomimetic intoxication. Gaze palsies, confusion, and ataxia could be due to thiamine deficiency leading to Wernicke's encephalopathy. Nystagmus occurs in PCP intoxication. Physical examination can detect fresh needle marks, recent alcohol intake, or nasal irritation from cocaine or inhalant abuse. Of course, patients frequently have comorbid medical and neurological conditions that affect mental and physical status, such as AIDS dementia, seizures, head trauma, and infections, and these conditions should be considered in diagnosis of the disorder and care of the patient.

Markedly altered mental status, evidence of recent substance abuse, and reliable corroborating history can aid in distinguishing between withdrawal, chronic organicity, and functional diagnoses. Diagnosis may be delayed or provisional in patients with a known chronic substance abuse history, unreliable recent history, and history of major psychiatric symptoms. Longstanding organicity can confound diagnosis when it has not been previously noted. Alcohol dementia and postconcussive head syndromes can sensitize the brain to react to minor substance abuse with dramatic and unpredictable results. In such patients, many things are ongoing concurrently. It is important to provide a safe environment, to protect the patient and others from harm, and to ensure basic airway, respiratory, and cardiac support until a basic diagnostic workup is completed.

Countertransference and Diagnosis

SUD patients with histrionic, paranoid, borderline, or antisocial features may present with an exacerbation of primitive defenses (e.g., projection, projective identification, and splitting during intoxication). These patients may become belligerent, distrustful, unappreciative, uncooperative, or violent, making management and history-taking difficult. Due to the strong countertransference such patients evoke, inappropriate diagnostic and treatment decisions may ensue. Before making an unusual treatment decision or participating in uncharacteristic behavior with a patient, consultation with another expert may be helpful, and sometimes a team approach is especially helpful. Even a simple time-out for the therapist to collect thoughts and feelings may be helpful. The patient's feelings should not be ignored but used to help clarify diagnosis. Frequently, obnoxious, uncooperative, destructive behavior or apparent personality problems are time limited and related to a substance-induced state. They may reflect the patient's fear and low self-esteem. A totally uncooperative patient, if tolerated through acute intoxication, can have a dramatic and unexpected turnaround.

■ PSYCHIATRIC COMORBIDITY

The term *dual diagnosis patients* refers to patients who have a substance abuse disorder and another major psychiatric diagnosis. The connections between the two may be manifold (8). Major psychiatric disorders may precede the development of substance abuse, develop concurrently, or manifest secondarily. Psychiatric disorders may precipitate the onset or modify the course of a substance abuse disorder. Psychiatric disorders and substance abuse may present as independent conditions. Thus it is difficult at any one point in time to differentiate symptoms of withdrawal, intoxication, and secondary cognitive, affective, perceptual, or personality changes from underlying psychiatric disorders. Important tools in differential diagnosis include careful history-taking, urine screens, and determination of the course or sequence of symptoms. Information obtained from third parties, including family history, is critical.

Affective Disorders

Regardless of the patient's expectations or experiences of euphoria during chronic use, chronic major depression occurs late in the course of addiction. This may be the result of altered neurochemistry, hormonal or metabolic changes, chronic demoralization, grief from personal losses, or the result of stresses of the addiction lifestyle. Chronic heroin use often leads to lethargy and social withdrawal. Sustained alcohol use generally produces depression and anxiety, although brief periods of euphoria may still occur.

It is vital to differentiate between alcohol-induced depressive disorder and primary depressive disorder. According to a large-sample-size study, primary major depressive episodes are more likely to occur in female, Caucasian, and married patients who have experienced fewer drugs and less treatment for alcoholism, have attempted suicide, and have a close relative with a major mood disorder (9). Although the majority of alcoholics will not have an independent diagnosis of major depressive disorder, other less severe depressive disorders may persist in a large proportion of alcoholics after cessation of drinking. Drinking may be more of a problem during a hypomanic or manic phase of a bipolar disorder than during the depressed phase. In the majority of cases, depressive symptomatology subsides after 3–4 weeks of abstinence and usually needs no pharmacological intervention. Use of antidepressants is indicated after a drug-free period, and abstinence is required for efficacy. Untreated major depression in a primary alcoholic or secondary alcoholism in a primary depressive patient worsens prognosis.

There is considerable evidence that depression occurs more frequently in active opioid users and may subside with abstinence. Prevalence of major depression ranges from 17% to 30% in heroin addicts and is considerably greater among methadone users. Prevalence of affective disorders in substance abuse patients in general is as high as 60%. Many depressive episodes are mild, related to stress, and may be related to treatment-seeking. In a 2.5-year follow-up study, depression was found to be a poor prognostic sign except in cases of coexistent antisocial personality, in which depression improved prognosis (10).

Affective disorders have been reported to exist concurrently in 30% of cocaine addicts, with a significant proportion of these patients having bipolar disorder or cyclothymia. Bipolar patients in a manic phase may use cocaine to heighten feelings of grandiosity. The profound dysphoric mood related to cocaine binges will resolve in the majority of cocaine addicts. A minority of patients may have underlying unipolar or bipolar disorder, which needs to be treated separately. This abstinence dysphoria may be secondary to depletion of brain catecholamines (e.g., dopamine) or to alteration in neural receptors, which results in postsynaptic supersensitivity. Some workers suggest that comorbid cocaine abuse acts as a robust predictor of poor outcome among depressed alcoholics.

Substance Abuse and Psychosis

Psychotic symptomatology can result from the use of a wide range of psychoactive substances: alcohol, cocaine, PCP, hallucinogens, and inhalants. As noted previously, all abused substances have organic syndromes that mimic various functional psychiatric syndromes. Opioids, however, have shown some antipsychotic properties.

The relationship between schizophrenia and substance abuse is more complex. Various studies have shown that 50%–60% of schizophrenic patients and 60%–80% of bipolar patients abuse substances (11). The role of substance abuse in precipitating or altering the course of an underlying schizophrenic disorder is unclear. Substance abuse may exacerbate symptoms in well-controlled schizophrenic patients. Alcohol, marijuana, hallucinogen, or cocaine abuse may produce psychotic symptoms that persist only in vulnerable individuals. It may be that schizophrenic patients seek out certain types of drugs for self-medication and for self-treatment of medication side effects. Patients with schizophrenia also use tobacco and caffeine more often than control subjects without schizophrenia. Tobacco use has been associated with lowering of blood levels of neuroleptics and leads to a need for higher-than-average doses of neuroleptics for symptom control. Schizophrenic patients may seek out drugs that increase the chance of precipitating psychotic episodes to feel a sense of mastery or experience merging. Schizophrenic patients may be treating dysphoria or negative symptoms of their disease and may use stimulants to allow them to feel more intensely. These patients may also be treating extrapyramidal or sedative side effects of neuroleptic medications. Schizophrenic patients who abuse stimulant drugs may also be treating an independent, underlying affective disorder. Substance abuse may provide the schizophrenic patient with the experience of control over unpredictable states of consciousness or may provide a strong identity as a substance abuser, which may be more palatable and perceived as being less stigmatic than having a major psychiatric disorder.

Anxiety Disorders

Generalized anxiety disorder, posttraumatic stress disorder (PTSD), panic disorder, and phobic disorder are overrepresented in substance abuse patients, especially alcoholics and sedative-hypnotic abusers. One study of alcoholics reported general anxiety disorder in 9% and phobias in 3%, which is significantly higher than in the general population (12). PTSD has been related to the high rates of alcoholism in Vietnam veterans who saw active duty. Panic disorder has been found in 5% of inpatient addicts (13). High dosages of benzodiazepines, up to 1,000 or 1,500 mg, have been reported in patients with underlying anxiety disorders. These patients are often very difficult to treat due to the complex interaction between the anxiety disorder and the substance abuse disorder. In treatment of addicted patients with anxiety disorders, benzodiazepines should be avoided if possible. Specific treatment of the underlying anxiety disorder may include typical and low-dose atypical antipsychotics, antidepressants, monoamine oxidase inhibitors, buspirone, gabapentin, or propranolol (see Chapter 8, Treatment Approaches for Substance Use Disorders).

Neuropsychiatric Impairment

Chronic abuse of alcohol, sedatives, and inhalants has been well correlated with chronic brain damage and neuropsychological impairment. These impairments may be gross, as evidenced in alcohol dementia or Korsakoff's syndrome, or relatively mild and detected only by neuropsychological testing. Cognitive impairment may be short-lived and recede after 3–4 weeks of abstinence, improve gradually over several months or years of abstinence, or be permanent. The damage caused by alcohol to brain tissue has been chronicled by abnormal computed tomography scan findings (cortical atrophy, which may reverse as well; see Chapter 6, Laboratory Findings and Diagnostic Instruments), altered EEG (decreased alpha activity), and altered evoked potential results (decreased P3 component). In the case of benzodiazepine abuse, however, the cognitive impairment may be reversible (14).

■ REFERENCES

1. American Psychiatric Association: Diagnostic and Statistical Manual of Mental Disorders, 4th Edition, Text Revision. Washington, DC, American Psychiatric Association, 2000

2. Spitzer RL, Williams JBW, Gibbon M: Structured Clinical Interview for DSM-IV. New York, New York State Psychiatric Institute, Biometrics Research, 1995

3. Schuckit MA, Smith TL, Daeppen JB, et al: Clinical relevance of the distinction between alcohol dependence with and without a physiological component. Am J Psychiatry 155:733–740, 1998

4. Nace E: Alcohol, in Clinical Textbook of Addictive Disorders, 2nd Edition. Edited by Frances RJ, Miller SI. New York, Guilford, 1998

5. Karan LD, Haller DH, Schnoll SH: Cocaine and stimulants, in Clinical Textbook of Addictive Disorders, 2nd Edition. Edited by Frances RJ, Miller SI. New York, Guilford, 1998

6. Flaum M, Schultz SK: When does amphetamine-induced psychosis become schizophrenia? Am J Psychiatry 153:812–815, 1996

7. Centers for Disease Control: Gamma-hydroxybutyrate use: NY and TX, 1995–1996. JAMA 277:1511, 1997

8. Vaillant GE: Is alcoholism more often the cause or result of depression? Harv Rev Psychiatry 1:94–99, 1993

9. Schuckit MA, Tipp JE, Bergman M, et al: Comparison of induced and independent major depressive disorders in 2,945 alcoholics. Am J Psychiatry 154:948–957, 1997

10. Brooner RK, King VL, Kidorf M, et al: Psychiatric and substance use comorbidity among treatment seeking opioid abusers. Arch Gen Psychiatry 54:71–80, 1997

11. Schneier FR, Siris SG: A review of psychoactive substance use and abuse in schizophrenia: patterns of drug choice. J Nerv Ment Dis 175:641, 1987

12. Ross HE, Glaser FB, Germanson T: The prevalence of psychiatric disorders in patients with alcohol and other drug problems. Arch Gen Psychiatry 45:1023–1031, 1988

13. Kushner MG, Sher KJ, Beitman BD: The relation between alcohol problems and the anxiety disorders. Am J Psychiatry 147:685–695, 1990

14. Salzman C, Fisher J, Nobel K, et al: Cognitive improvement following benzodiazepine discontinuation in elderly nursing home residents. Int J Geriatr Psychiatry 7:89–93, 1992

5

THE FRONT LINE
Detecting and Approaching Substance Abuse in the General Hospital and in the Workplace

■ THE GENERAL HOSPITAL

It has been estimated that 25%–50% of general hospital admissions are related to complications of substance use (1). A high level of suspicion may help the health care provider to detect a hidden substance use disorder (SUD). There may be further advantages in confronting the addictive process during a medical crisis when denial may be lessened or can be easily confronted by irrefutable medical evidence. Alcoholism may be diagnosed by associated medical problems, such as liver disease, pancreatitis, anemia, certain types of pneumonia, delirium, dementia, gastric ulcers, esophageal varices, tuberculosis, or symptoms that mimic psychiatric syndromes.

Admission Workup

In the general hospital setting, detailed alcohol and substance use histories should be taken on admission from every patient. Information should be gathered in a straightforward manner in concert with the rest of the medical history. When substance use problems do exist, the patient's answers may be vague, evasive, or aggressively defensive. In early abuse patterns, some patients may be surprised by the connection between their substance use and their current medical problems. Health professionals should be knowledgeable about the components of a basic alcohol and substance use history (Table 5–1). Because of the patient's possible denial, resistance, organicity, and psychiatric symptoms, a consultation with an addiction specialist may be helpful in making a diagnosis. Third-party sources such as family or friends may be necessary to obtain crucial information. For example, additional corroboration was necessary in the assessment of prior alcohol abuse in a man who had been admitted for routine surgery and denied alcohol abuse on admission but appeared to be in early delirium tremens two days later. The psychoactive substance abuse history should be a systematic review of all the major drug classes. Often patients will not consider a particular substance to be a drug. For example, a 30-year-old woman who had been smoking marijuana every day since college did not consider marijuana a drug. Asking her if she abused drugs seemed to her a pejorative question. She did not offer the desired information due to a lack of knowledge and her particular view of the stigma of drug abuse.

TABLE 5–1.   **Components of a basic alcohol and substance use history**

Chief complaint
Current medical signs and symptoms
Substance abuse review of systems for all substances of abuse
Dates of first use, regular use, longest period of sobriety and overall life condition during sobriety, pattern, amount, frequency, time of last use, route of administration, circumstances of use, reactions to use
Medical history, medications, HIV and TB status
History of past substance abuse treatment, response to treatment, history of complications secondary to substances
Psychiatric history
Family history of psychiatric disease and substance use
Legal history
Object relations history
Personal and social history
Review of collected data (chart, family, primary care physician)

Specific Substance History-Taking

Experience with drug classes such as alcohol, opioids, cocaine or other stimulants, tranquilizers, hallucinogens, marijuana, inhalants, and over-the-counter medication should be systematically ascertained. Use and possible abuse of prescription medications should be covered. The history should include the type of liquor or specific drug, amount, pattern or frequency of use, and time of last use. The later historical information may be very important in distinguishing various organic mental states. The route of administration (oral, intravenous, or pulmonary inhalation) may have important health consequences. For example, HIV screening should be done on the vast majority of intravenous drug addicts who present for admission in the general hospital setting. If alcohol abuse is suspected, symptoms of physical dependence must be actively pursued. Missing such information can be life threatening.

A history of early-morning tremors or shakes, a subjective need for a drink to calm the nerves, elevated pulse and blood pressure, or a known history of alcohol-related seizures or delirium tremens should signal the need for pharmacological detoxification. Polysubstance abuse may mask underlying physical dependence on one prominent psychoactive substance (e.g., opioids in speed balling [mixing cocaine and heroin] or hits [combined use of heroin and cocaine], or alcohol dependence secondary to cocaine addiction). Question the patient about past hospitalization for motor vehicle accidents, accidental injuries, or substance-related violence in addition to any history of treatment for alcohol or other substance abuse problems.

■ PSYCHIATRIC CONSULTATION TO GENERAL FLOORS AND THE EMERGENCY DEPARTMENT

The general hospital staff may request psychiatric consultations for straightforward evaluation such as substance abuse evaluation or for more cryptic evaluations of organicity, mood disorders, or acting-out behavior. Requests may be for help in treating overdose and withdrawal, making an initial diagnosis, engaging patients in the therapeutic process, evaluating pain medications, treating trauma and burn patients and pregnant substance abusers, and making assessments for transplant. Often the house staff perceives the patients who need psychiatric consultation as being manipulative, demanding, and unappreciative, and often, in reality, they can present as such. It is important not to disavow the staff's real feelings but to provide a framework of understanding of the addictive process that can make these feelings meaningful and tolerable. Clinicians may find it intolerable when these negative feelings surface; few people go into medicine to dislike their patients. The clinician's realization of feelings induced by patients is not only at times diagnostic, but it may also relieve the guilt of experiencing retaliatory fantasies. In affective illnesses, the presence of overwhelming affects may focus attention away from a concomitant addictive process. In cases of organicity, important historical information may simply be forgotten. Table 5–2 offers general guidelines for approaching this patient population.

Each consultation request should be reviewed in an attempt to most clearly ascertain the nature of the request. Frequently, this requires a call to the referring physician. Questions of confidenti-

---

TABLE 5–2. **General considerations in the approach to psychiatric consultation**

Have a high suspicion for drug abuse and get collected data

Obtain serum and urine toxicology screens as soon as possible after admission

Know general principles of detoxification and its differential therapeutics

Realize that detoxification often needs to be tailored to individual medical patients

Recall that when treating polysubstance dependence, sedative withdrawal occurs first

Use challenge tests or estimate conservatively when considering initial detoxification dose

Recognize drug-drug interactions and effects of medications on mental status exam

Always differentiate psychopathology, substance-induced disorders, and medical disorders

---

ality may arise with patients regarding their substance abuse. Generally, confidentiality should be discussed and handled appropriately. Because honesty is one of the core treatment tools in an addictive disease process, conspiracies or secrets regarding substance abuse are not advisable.

Assessing the Chart

As a consultant, reviewing the medical chart in detail is essential, not only to obtain important information about signs and symptoms from admission, third-party statements, and the mental status of the patient, but also to compile divergent clues of substance abuse in a fresh manner. Pertinent laboratory work, X rays, electroencephalograms, computed tomography scans, and so forth, should be reviewed. Suggestions for additional laboratory work (e.g., magnesium levels in a patient with a history of delirium tremens) should be made.

The Interview

If the consult request asks for assessment of a substance abuse problem, this should be clearly stated to the patient early in the interview. The referring physician can be asked to join the interview if it seems appropriate. In writing up findings, it is best to briefly note the patient's impressions of the reason for the consultation and his or her identifying information, a brief synopsis of the present illness, and the patient's history, medical complications, medications, and mental status. The impressions and recommendations should be prominent and the focus of the consult. Often this record is the only one read.

Treatment Planning

Specific recommendations for treatment range from outpatient substance abuse treatment to no further intervention, to inpatient substance abuse or psychiatric treatment. Often active treatment must be postponed until the acute medical problems are stabilized. For patients showing early abuse patterns, simple counseling, education, and appropriate reassurance may be all that is necessary. If the patient does not have marked medical or psychiatric complications, is motivated, and has a less serious abuse pattern and little prior treatment exposure, outpatient referral is preferable. Inpatient psychiatric treatment may be indicated when major psychiatric illnesses need to be treated (psychosis, major depression) or with suicidal or homicidal ideation. Many units for mentally ill chemical-abusing patients have been created to treat the substance abuser having major psychiatric problems. Transfer to an inpatient rehabilitation unit, when indicated, should be through a direct transfer from the hospital to the treatment facility. All detoxification regimens should be clearly and explicitly spelled out. It may be necessary to work with the treatment staff to modify regimens in case of medical complications, such as liver or renal disease.

Additional Treatment Issues

It is important to realize that abstinence in itself is not evidence of satisfactory treatment; a patient can be free of drug or alcohol use or craving while in the hospital and quickly return to active use on discharge. Family and individual education about substance abuse and assessment of the meaning of drugs or alcohol use in that person's life can begin in the hospital. Drug urine screens or alcohol Breathalyzer tests may need to be obtained for general hospital inpatients. Occasionally, patients will find methods to use substances even while in the hospital. These patients should be transferred to locked units, where articles and people entering can be monitored for contraband. Early confrontation of continuing alcohol or drug use may clear up complicated diagnostic pictures.

Making the Referral

It is often best that the patient make the initial call to initiate treatment. It is also important that all calls be made while in the hospital setting and that appointments are set before discharge. In cases where substance abuse treatment facilities are connected with the general hospital, in-house contact is advised, as well as attendance at in-house meetings, such as those of Alcoholics Anonymous, when feasible.

Drug Interactions

Special attention to drug interactions is necessary in the general hospital setting. When first admitted, patients may have psychoactive drugs in their system that will adversely interact with prescribed medications. Alcohol interacts with other medications in various ways (Table 5–3). One interesting and important way in which it does so is by its bimodal effect on the cytochrome P450 system. Initially alcohol can inhibit the metabolism of other drugs, thus increasing serum levels of oral anticoagulants, diazepam, and phenytoin. But after chronic use, alcohol can induce cytochrome P450 enzymes, leading to decreased levels of these medications. Thorazine, chloral hydrate, and cimetidine all inhibit alcohol dehydrogenase. Finally, alcohol increases the absorption of diazepam and the potency of all CNS depressants.

TABLE 5–3.	**Medications and interactions with alcohol**
Disulfiram	Flushing, diaphoresis, vomiting, confusion
Oral anticoagulants	Increased effect with acute intoxication, decreased effect after chronic use
Antimicrobials	Minor Antabuse reaction
Sedatives, hypnotics, narcotics, antihistamines	Increased central nervous system depression
Diazepam	Increased absorption
Phenytoin	Increased anticonvulsant effect with acute intoxication; alcohol intoxication or withdrawal may lower seizure threshold after chronic alcohol abuse
Salicylates	Gastrointestinal bleeding
Chlorpromazine	Increased levels of alcohol, lowered seizure threshold
Monoamine oxide inhibitors	Adverse reactions to tyramine in some alcoholic beverages

Management of Pain

Iatrogenic contributions to addiction are a major concern in treating substance abuse patients in the general hospital setting. These contributions are most notable in intravenous drug addicts for whom pain medication is required. Many staff members are trained to be very cautious and suspicious when prescribing pain medication for these patients. Excessive caution can lead to undermedication. These patients may present with low frustration tolerance, anxiety, demanding behavior, and manipulation. It must be stressed, however, that these patients do experience pain; if too much rage and anger are evoked in the staff, treatment personnel may be unconsciously driven to punish offensive patients by undermedicating them. In certain individuals, larger than usual doses of pain medications are indicated because of tolerance. Each patient should be evaluated carefully, taking into account history, pattern of abuse, personality, and physical pathology. When the concerns and requests of substance abuse patients are categorically dismissed, serious prejudicial attitudes may be evident. In some cases, affected staff should remove themselves from the patient's care before a spiral develops that will end in the abandonment of the patient.

Chronic pain patients have a high profile for abusing drugs. The concept of *pain behavior* has been recognized. "Madison" is the acronym for a test that scores pain behavior and includes assessment of such factors as variable pain patterns, strong needs to authenticate the pain, denial of emotional problems, pain associated with interpersonal relationships, idealization then devaluation of doctors, a feeling of being unique, and the feeling that nothing helps (2). Maintaining continuity of care and promoting realistic expectations are prominent treatment goals. It is necessary to avoid intramuscular medication and as-needed dose scheduling and to ensure adequate coverage (i.e., selection of medications that have adequate half-lives for dosage scheduling, appropriate administration, and the appropriate medication for the type of pain) (2).

Burn Patients

Use of alcohol and other substances is a risk factor for burns. And preburn use of these substances implies a worse prognosis for the burn patient: alcohol is an independent predictor of death in such patients (3). Burn patients who use alcohol or other substances require important attention from psychiatric and substance use standpoints both in coping with present loss and in treatment planning for the future.

Organ Transplants

Increasing numbers of organ transplants will be performed in the future. Mental health personnel will be asked to assess patients' psychological readiness to receive such transplants. In developing criteria for eligibility for heart or liver transplants, alcoholism must be considered a complicating factor. Active alcoholism has been a contraindication for liver transplantation, although controversy surrounds this issue. Evaluation of recovering alcoholics is complicated. Up to half of all cases of hepatic failure in the United States are due to alcohol. Care must be taken not to discriminate against a stable recovering alcoholic who may well be a good candidate to receive a transplant. The fear of relapse, which would undermine the benefits of this treatment, is a consideration; however, careful evaluation and application of certain criteria may diminish this risk. Such criteria might include at least 6 months of sobriety from alcohol, no other active substance abuse, and good family support. The recovering alcoholic may be able to be evaluated in line with other candidates. In fact, there is evidence that organ and patient survival rates among selected recovering alcoholics who receive organ transplants are as good as those for patients who receive transplants for non-alcohol-related diseases (4).

■ THE WORKPLACE

Increasingly since the 1970s, the military, a large number of major corporations, and insurance carriers have recognized the value of early identification and evaluation of chemical dependency problems and have offered chemically dependent employees opportunities for treatment and assistance. Approximately 10,000 employee assistance programs (EAPs) have helped to reduce costs associated with increased absenteeism and medical claims due to substance abuse. Many corporations have also established general fitness and wellness programs, which emphasize exercise, weight control, cessation of smoking, stress reduction, and detection of warning signs of illness. In addition to liability due to accidents, costly mistakes, and morale problems affecting co-workers of a troubled employee, considerable costs are incurred by firing, hiring, and retraining employees. The hidden benefits of rehabilitation programs are not lost on administrators concerned with cost-effectiveness. In addition to retaining valuable employees, the corporations find that these programs reduce union pressure that could occur from firing employees whose job performances do not improve because they fail to follow through with treatment. Unions have recognized the value of the health benefits associated with EAPs as a way of improving labor-management relations. Increasingly, unions are pressing to make the programs available to family members as part of benefit packages.

Case Finding at the Workplace

In our culture, the greatest pressure that leads those with SUDs to accept treatment occurs in the workplace. Usually those with SUDs do not seek help until a crisis has occurred somewhere in their lives. Frequently, people will not seek treatment until their jobs are threatened, even though they may have marital, medical, or other problems resulting from substance abuse. Fellow employees and managers may be overprotective of a troubled employee and wait until a crisis occurs that leads to firing. It is helpful to teach supervisors that early recognition of job performance problems and referral to an EAP for evaluation can result in job protection and improved health. SUD patients who still have jobs and marriages intact have the best prognosis.

The Employee Assistance Program Model

Most EAPs have both voluntary and mandatory portals of entry. Once workers see that the program has been successful for others, many volunteer for treatment; the ratio of volunteer to compulsory referrals often exceeds 10:1. EAPs are most often run by the company with in-house counselors and are connected to personnel or medical departments. The employee can approach the EAP representative voluntarily and confidentially before major job problems have arisen. Supervisors, union representatives, and employees are given educational materials on descriptions of the program and the warning signs of work performance problems. Supervisors document work-related problems and are encouraged not to make a diagnosis or speculate on the specific diagnosis of an employee's work problems. Supervisors suggest a meeting with the EAP counselor and, if the job is at stake, may make a mandatory referral to the EAP counselor. The employee who has had a documented history of work-related problems may face a choice between acceptance of the referral and job action. This basically provides the employee with another opportunity to improve work performance with the addition of treatment. Information obtained during the process is not shared with the supervisor and is kept confidential. Ultimate job action depends on job performance rather than on the recommendation of either the EAP counselor or the treatment resource. Confidentiality is essential to any successful EAP. Companies have found that it is better to treat and retain recovering SUD patients than to have employees with undetected problems.

The EAP model has evolved somewhat during the 1990s. Previously the typical EAP was staffed by recovering, nonclinical personnel, and the EAP office had little or no visibility with senior leadership, which created a less than ideal relationship with external mental health and substance abuse practitioners because the structure was reactive rather than proactive. Corporations such as Hughes Electronics pride themselves in now having EAPs that are adapting to the need for integrated and managed health care: they are increasingly proactive, having so-called stress debriefing after critical incidents and workplace violence teams. Unfortunately, human resources managers restrict substance abuse service coverage to a great extent. Nonetheless, the workplace's attention to SUDs will continue to evolve.

Job Impairment

Employees may experience either problems related to the use of substances on the job or the effects of chronic abuse that occurs after work hours. Disability may include medical, psychiatric, and social consequences of chronic use. Off-hours drinking and substance abuse can contribute to hangovers, withdrawal symptoms, absenteeism, medical and psychiatric complications, and preoccupation with obtaining or using the substances, all of which can interfere with concentration on the job. Off-duty problems such as charges of driving while intoxicated or drug possession are an embarrassment to a company, and legal and illegal off-hours substance abuse can affect employee morale. Use of substances can contribute to corruption and white-collar crime. Military plane crashes have been found to be associated with use of marijuana, alcohol, and other substances by either ground or air crews. Physician impairment is a major problem in the medical profession, and physician's health programs have been established in 50 states. Companies tend to be more punitive for other substance abuse than for alcohol abuse. Many companies will require a ''Ulysses'' contract from substance abusers, which provides that the employee abstain from drugs and if the employee returns to the habit, that the employer be notified and employment be terminated. A better understanding of prevailing negative attitudes regarding those with SUDs and of the particular problems and needs of corporations that employ them will be important. The growing concern of corporate benefits departments under pressure to require cost-effectiveness is likely to lead to improvement and sharpening of measurable treatment goals.

■ REFERENCES

1. Moore RD, Bone LR, Geller G, et al: Prevalence, detection, and treatment of alcoholism in hospitalized patients. JAMA 261:403–407, 1989
2. Bouckoms A, Hackett TP: Pain patients, in MGH Handbook of General Hospital Psychiatry, 4th Edition. Edited by Cassem NH. St. Louis, MO, Mosby-Yearbook Publishing, 1997, pp 367–415
3. McGill V, Kowal-Vern A, Fisher SG: The impact of substance use on mortality and morbidity from thermal injury. J Trauma 38:931–934, 1995
4. Berlakovich GA, Steininger R, Herbst F, et al: Efficacy of liver transplantation for alcoholic cirrhosis with respect to recidivism and compliance. Transplantation 58:560–565, 1994

6

LABORATORY FINDINGS AND DIAGNOSTIC INSTRUMENTS

■ RATIONALE FOR TESTING

The following are valid reasons for drug testing:

- Poor drug histories
- Clinical correlations
- Differential diagnosis
- Routine follow-up
- Assessment
- Forensic needs
- Athletics issues
- Public safety
- Relapse detection
- Deterrence through routine testing

■ LABORATORY FINDINGS: URINE AND BLOOD SCREENS

In the absence of a clear history of a substance use disorder (SUD), several physical signs and laboratory test results may indicate a patient's primary substance abuse disorder. Vital sign changes, agitation, irritability or unpredictable behavior, needle marks or scars, and evidence of unexplained trauma may all signal substance abuse. Inadequate management of pain with unusual analgesic dosages and unexpected elevated blood levels of commonly abused substances (e.g., alcohol) without obvious intoxication may also signal drug or alcohol tolerance and addiction.

The importance of analysis of urine and blood levels for appropriate substances cannot be overstressed as a means to screen and provide collateral evidence for substance abuse problems. The sensitivity and accuracy of blood and urine screening has improved with the addition of gas chromatography to more routine screening techniques. A general toxicology screen includes a blood alcohol level (BAL) test.

■ SELECTION OF TOXICOLOGICAL TESTS AND PHARMACOKINETICS

There are five points to consider when choosing a test:

1. What to sample
2. Half-life of the suspected substance
3. Significance of biotransformation of the suspected substance
4. Sensitivity and specificity of the test
5. Cost

Knowledge of the half-life of various drug doses helps in analyzing the results. For example, the half-life of 4 ounces of orally administered ethyl alcohol will be 1–2 hours. A BAL of 200 mg/dL indicates recent heavy alcohol intake and most likely current intoxication. A negative paper chromatography drug screen for cocaine in a man admitted for a 2-day history of paranoid, delusional behavior does not rule out abuse because cocaine has a relatively short half-life (it clears in 24–36 hours) and because paper chromatography has a low sensitivity (1). Marijuana, which is highly fat soluble, has a relatively long half-life and can be detected in the urine of heavy users up to 3 weeks after the last use.

Urine Drug Screens

Urine drug screen results usually are reported as either positive or negative for any particular drug. Most routine urine screens cover the major drugs of abuse. Specificity and sensitivity are lower with thin-layer chromatography and immunoassay techniques. More sophisticated and sensitive quantitative testing with gas chromatography–mass spectrometry (GC-MS) can be done later for certain drugs (e.g., marijuana) if urine from the original sample tests positive. The results of urine drug screens generally are not useful in court because they do not answer the question of degree of intoxication. For general hospital purposes, urine drug screens are imperative in certain situations. In cases of unknown coma, of atypical psychiatric presentations, or with agitated and confused patients with known drug histories or physical evidence of substance abuse, urine drug screening should be routine. In high-risk populations or areas where drugs may be epidemic (e.g., certain inner-city general hospitals), urine drug screening should be routinely done for psychiatric admissions. In order to ensure the validity and reliability of urine screen results, direct observation of voiding may be indicated. Finally, it should be noted that morning urine samples are often contaminated and should be avoided if possible.

Blood Screening Tests

Suspicion of alcoholism or substance abuse may be heightened with corroborating laboratory evidence from blood studies (Table 6–1), and this evidence is often useful in forensic cases. Elevated mean corpuscular volume (MCV) and liver function tests with el-

---

TABLE 6–1. **Laboratory findings associated with alcohol abuse**

Blood alcohol level
Positive Breathalyzer results
Elevated MCV
Elevated SGOT, SGPT, LDH levels
Elevated GGT levels (particularly sensitive)
Decreased albumin, B_{12}, folic acid
Increased uric acid, elevated amylase, and evidence of bone marrow suppression

---

evated levels of compounds such as serum glutamic-oxaloacetic transaminase (SGOT), also known as aspartate transaminase (AST), serum glutamic-pyruvic transaminase (SGPT), also known as alanine transaminase (ALT), and lactate dehydrogenase (LDH) may be a sign of alcohol abuse. Elevated levels of serum gamma-glutamyl transpeptidase (SGGT), a measure of liver enzyme induction, is a particularly sensitive indicator of possible alcoholic liver disease. More than 70% of those who drink heavily have an elevated level of gamma-glutamyltransferase (GGT) (>40 units/L). Active alcoholics have a 4-fold to 10-fold higher rate of abnormal GGT levels than when they are abstinent. GGT as an indicator of heavy alcohol consumption has a sensitivity of 70% and a specificity of 90%. The AST level is elevated (>45 units/L) in 30%–60% of alcoholics, with a sensitivity of 80%. Irwin et al. reported preliminary evidence that increases of 20% for GGT levels and 50% for AST levels over baseline abstinence are possible indicators of heavy drinking even if the increased values fall within the normal range and therefore may be an indicator of relapse (2).

Increased MCV, a measure of red blood cell size (>95 μm^3 in males, 100 μm^3 in females), is found with certain nutritional deficiencies (e.g., folate or B_{12}) or can be associated with the direct effect of alcohol on bone marrow cell production. Increased MCV is found in 45%–90% of alcoholics, whereas only 1%–5% of non-alcoholics demonstrate elevated MCV (3).

Attempts are being made to develop laboratory profiles that will serve as better markers for early detection of alcohol abuse. For example, the combination of abnormal GGT levels and abnormal MCV identifies 90% of alcoholics in the general medical population compared to 70%–80% when MCV or GGT levels are used alone (4). Unfortunately, at this time, these panels have false-negative and false-positive results that are unacceptable for clinical use other than screening. Finally, decreased serum albumin, B_{12}, or folate levels may be evidence of prolonged malnutrition secondary to alcohol or substance abuse. Positive tests for hepatitis B, HIV, and bacteremia may indicate past or present intravenous substance use. Laboratory findings consistent with pancreatitis, hepatitis, bone marrow suppression, or certain types of infection indicate alcoholism. In coming years the detection of carbohydrate-deficient transferrin (CDT) will be increasingly important in detecting relapse and heavy alcohol use. Although the test is available in many U.S. research laboratories, there has not been widespread clinical use of it to this point. This is unfortunate because the CDT test is superior to the SGGT test in detecting relapse or recent heavy use (5).

Other Studies

Sweat, hair, and saliva have been increasingly used as laboratory specimens to test for substance use disorders, but their clinical reliability remains unknown. Breathalyzer tests are simple, do not require an invasive procedure, provide immediate results, and are widely used. Liver, spleen, and brain scans and electroencephalograms may also be useful in the diagnosis of substance abuse.

■ INTERPRETING TEST RESULTS

Qualitative presence of drugs indicates prior exposure but perhaps not current intoxication or impairment. To help clarify the situation consider the following questions: What method of testing was used? Did the assay analyze for the drug, the metabolite, or both? What was the cutoff threshold (call the lab if unclear)? Was the time the sample was taken close to the time of exposure?

When considering the possibility of a false-positive result, first determine whether it is possible. A false positive is almost impossible when using thin-layer chromatography (TLC) because it is a highly specific method, although poorly sensitive, for both drugs and their metabolites, and because color dyes increase specificity. In radioimmunoassays (RIAs) or enzyme-multiplied immunoassay technique (EMIT), two sensitive tests, chemically similar compounds may cross-react, producing false positives. Furthermore, because each antibody has a particular affinity, the specificity of each test should be evaluated. Immunoassays can be confirmed by chromatography and vice versa.

False-negative results occur more easily than false-positive results. Remember that once a specimen tests negative it is not tested further. Yet negative TLC results are not conclusive. Cutoffs may be too high for RIAs or enzyme immunoassays. When the suspicion for use is strong, the clinician should repeat the test and consult the laboratory for more sensitive drug screening procedures such as GC-MS.

■ DIAGNOSTIC INSTRUMENTS

Attempts at defining accurate psychological makeups for those who abuse alcohol and other substances generally have failed. Early psychodynamic theorists described addictive behavior as related to oral regressive defense mechanisms. More recently, theorists have discussed ego disturbances, difficulty with affect regulation, and defective self-care mechanisms. Pathological dependency, feelings of inadequacy, and counterdependency feelings of bravado have been described.

Cognitive theorists have posited psychoactive substance abuse participation as involving tension and stress reduction, positive expectancy of mood elevation, and increased perception of self-adequacy. Additional psychiatric diagnoses have been described in 50% of alcoholics and cocaine abusers and in up to 93% of intravenous heroin abusers. No single alcohol or substance abuse personality has proven to be etiological.

Diagnostic Research Instruments

The need for better standardized diagnostic research instruments in psychiatry has produced structured interviews that have been helpful in identifying alcoholism in large epidemiological studies. These instruments are also used to identify other psychiatric diagnoses. The Schedule for Affective Disorders, based on the Research Diagnostic Criteria (RDC), is a forerunner to the Diagnostic Instrument Schedule (DIS). The DIS is based on DSM-IV criteria and is designed as an instrument that can be administered by trained lay interviewers. The Structured Clinical Interview for DSM-IV is a more recent structured interview based on the DSM-IV criteria that also has a capability to make DSM-IV personality disorder diagnoses. These instruments have proven to be fairly reliable in establishing DSM-IV and RDC psychoactive substance abuse diagnoses. However, within the psychoactive substance abuse population, problems may exist in assessing other psychiatric diagnoses with these instruments. The anxiety, antisocial, and depression sections may be less useful in the psychoactive substance abuse population.

There are several instruments designed for research purposes that finely measure attributes of alcohol abuse. The Alcohol Use Inventory (AUI) (6) is a 17-item, self-administered questionnaire that reflects 1) the perceived benefits of alcohol, 2) the problems concomitant to alcohol use, 3) the disruptive consequences of drinking, and 4) the patient's concern about the use of alcohol and the extent to which the patient acknowledges having a drinking problem.

Dimensional Scales

Dimensional personality profile scales such as the Minnesota Multiphasic Personality Inventory (MMPI) and the Hopkins Symptom Checklist–90 have been useful in substance abuse populations. In the hands of a skilled interpreter, common findings of elevated hysteria, paranoia, antisocial, and depression subscale results can augment initial clinical impressions. A markedly elevated schizophrenia scale result or evidence of gender identity confusion may occasionally be expected. Profiles may indicate that the patient is dissimulating to fake good or bad results. Although limited to augmentation of a good clinical diagnostic interview, the MMPI may be most useful for charting improvement over time. Due to the time-limited organic effects of alcohol, patients' symptoms frequently begin to clear after 3 or 4 weeks of abstinence, and this is reflected in the test. Personality subscale results may improve as the acquired substance abuse–related personality attributes begin to clear. Conversely, serious psychiatric problems may also be un-

TABLE 6–2. **The Michigan Alcoholism Screening Test (MAST)**

Points	Question	Yes	No
(0)	0. Do you enjoy a drink now and then?		
(2)	1. Do you feel you are a normal drinker? (By normal we mean you drink less than or as much as most other people.) [Negative response is alcoholic response]		
(2)	2. Have you ever awakened the morning after some drinking the night before and found that you could not remember a part of the evening?		
(1)	3. Does you wife, husband, parent, or other near relative ever worry or complain about your drinking?		
(2)	4. Can you stop drinking without a struggle after one or two drinks? [Negative response is alcoholic response]		
(1)	5. Do you ever feel guilty about your drinking?		
(2)	6. Do friends or relatives think you are a normal drinker? [Negative response is alcoholic response]		
(0)	7. Do you ever try to limit your drinking to certain times of the day or to certain places?		
(2)	8. Are you always able to stop drinking when you want to? [Negative response is alcoholic response]		
(2)	9. Have you ever attended a meeting of Alcoholics Anonymous?		
(1)	10. Have you gotten into physical fights when drinking?		
(2)	11. Has your drinking ever created problems between you and your wife, husband, a parent, or other relative?		
(2)	12. Has your wife or husband (or other family members) ever gone to anyone for help about your drinking?		

(2) 13. Have you ever lost friends because of your drinking?

(2) 14. Have you ever gotten into trouble at work or school because of drinking?

(2) 15. Have you ever lost a job because of drinking?

(2) 16. Have you ever neglected your obligations, your family, or your work for 2 or more days in a row because you were drinking?

(1) 17. Do you drink before noon fairly often?

(2) 18. Have you ever been told you have liver trouble? Cirrhosis?

(2) *19. After heavy drinking, have you ever had delirium tremens (d.t.'s), severe shaking, or heard voices or seen things that really were not there?

(5) 20. Have you ever gone to anyone for help about your drinking?

(5) 21. Have you ever been in a hospital because of drinking?

(2) 22. Have you ever been a patient in a psychiatric hospital or on a psychiatric ward of a general iospital where drinking was part of the problem that resulted in hospitalization?

(2) 23. Have you ever been seen at a psychiatric or mental health clinic or gone to any doctor, social worker, or clergyman for help with any emotional problem where drinking was part of the problem?

(2) **24. Have you ever been arrested for drunk driving, driving while intoxicated, or driving under the influence of alcoholic beverages? (If YES, how many times? _____)

(2) **25. Have you ever been arrested or taken into custody—even for a few hours—because of other drunk behavior? (If YES, how many times? _____)

*Five points for d.t.'s   **Two points for each arrest

Scoring system: In general, 5 points or more would place the subject in an "alcoholic" category, 4 points would suggest alcoholism, 3 points or less would indicate the subject is not alcoholic.

Note. The MAST scoring system is very sensitive at the 5-point level and indicates more people to be alcoholics than anticipated. However, because it is a screening test, it should be sensitive at its lower levels.

Source. Reprinted from Selzer ML: "The Michigan Alcoholism Screening Test: The Quest for a New Diagnostic Instrument." *American Journal of Psychiatry* 127:1653–1658, 1971. Used with permission. Copyright American Psychiatric Association 1971.

masked following drug removal. Frequently, damage to personality structure improves, but recovery may not be total. The Mac-Andrews scale is a subset scale of the MMPI that has been widely used for identifying alcoholics. The MacAndrews scale is a 48-question true-false scale that can correctly identify 82% of alcoholics. Although this scale has shown promise, recent studies have highlighted some of its limitations in the general medical population.

Diagnostic Screening Devices

There are several instruments designed to measure various aspects of alcohol and other substance abuse. The majority of these instruments are not based on research criteria but have been found to be clinically useful in identifying psychoactive substance abuse. Two widely used screening tests for alcoholism are the Michigan Alcoholism Screening Test (MAST) (Table 6–2) and the CAGE Questionnaire (Table 6–3). These tests have the advantage of being self-administered, brief screens that can point the way for further study. The MAST is a 25-question form. The short MAST (SMAST) is a 13-item scale that correlates .90 with the MAST. The MAST has a test-retest reliability in excess of .85. The sensitivities of the MAST and of the SMAST are approximately .90 and .70, respectively. The proportion of nonalcoholics correctly identified as such averages .74 for the MAST. The MAST and SMAST tests screen for the major psychological, social, and physiological consequences of alcoholism. One new screening instrument for alcoholism, the TWEAK, has been found to be particularly helpful in screening women who drink (7).

Addiction Severity Index

The Addiction Severity Index (ASI) developed by McLellan et al. has proven to be a useful instrument for the substance abuse field, particularly regarding treatment outcome research. The ASI reaches a scale and scoring system for the severity of need

TABLE 6–3.	**CAGE screen for diagnosis of alcoholism**

"Have you ever?"

- C Thought you should CUT back on your drinking?
- A Felt ANNOYED by people criticizing your drinking?
- G Felt GUILTY or bad about your drinking?
- E Had a morning EYE OPENER to relieve hangover or nerves?

Score total positive responses: 2–3, high index of suspicion;
4, pathognomic

Source. Reprinted from Ewing JA: "Detecting Alcoholism: The CAGE Questionaire." *JAMA* 252:1905–1907, 1984. Used with permission. Copyrighted 1984, American Medical Association.

for treatment in seven major areas: medical status, employment-support status, drug use, alcohol use, legal status, family social relationships, and psychiatric status. This dimensional approach is most helpful in identifying treatment needs when attempting to match the patient with a specific tailored treatment. The instrument can be given by any trained person and takes approximately 50–60 minutes to administer. There is now also an ASI geared toward teenagers (9).

■ REFERENCES

1. Gold MS, Dackis CA: Role of the laboratory in the evaluation of suspected drug abuse. J Clin Psychiatry 47:17–23, 1986
2. Irwin M, Baird S, Smith TL, Schuckit M: Use of laboratory tests to monitor heavy drinking by alcoholic men discharged from a treatment program. Am J Psychiatry 145:595–599, 1988
3. Skinner M: Early identification of alcohol abuse. Can Med J 124:1279–1295, 1981
4. Lumeng L: New diagnostic markers of alcohol abuse. Hepatology 6:742–745, 1986
5. Schmidt LG, Schmidt K, Dufeu P, et al: Superiority of carbo-hydrate-deficient transferrin to gamma-glutamyltransferase in detecting relapse in alcoholism. Am J Psychiatry 154:75–80, 1997

6. Warberg K, Horn J: The Alcohol Use Inventory. Port Logan, CO, Multivariate Measurement Consultants, 1985
7. Russel M, Martier SS, Sokol RJ, et al: Screening for pregnancy risk-drinking: TWEAKING the tests. Alcohol Clin Exp Res 15:368, 1991
8. McLellan AT, Luborsky L, Woody GE, et al: Are the "addiction-related" problems of substance abusers really related? J Nerv Ment Dis 169:232–239, 1981
9. Kaminer Y, Bukstein O, Tarter RE: The Teen-Addiction Severity Index: rationale and reliability. International Journal of Addiction 26:219–226, 1991

7

NATURAL HISTORIES OF SUBSTANCE ABUSE

■ ALCOHOL

The signs and symptoms of alcoholism can be strikingly consistent among individuals whose disease has progressed to late stages. However, with the concept of case heterogeneity in mind, there appear to be subtypes of alcoholism that may present with different ages at onset, different underlying etiologies, different degrees of hereditary influence, different social and cultural backgrounds, and different natural outcomes. Vaillant has conducted one of the few prospective longitudinal studies of alcoholics (1). In his studies, many alcoholics continued to drink until death, some stopped drinking, and others showed a pattern of long abstinence followed by relapses. Nevertheless, some medical personnel have an unduly pessimistic view of the natural course of alcoholism and believe alcoholics will not get better with or without treatment. Family members may have unrealistically hopeful wishes and believe that the alcoholic will stop drinking in the near future without help. Large-scale outcome studies suggest that approximately 30% of alcoholics will at some point during the course of their illness achieve stable abstinence without any form of treatment (2). This percentage improves in some studies to approximately 70% with some form of treatment. Treatment could include professional treatment and/or self-help groups. Vaillant also described a series of natural healing forces (e.g., church involvement, fear of medical complications, fear of family loss) that may substitute for some aspects of formal treatment through the meeting of dependency needs.

Thus it is important to understand alcoholism as a disease that has many different patterns and is sometimes characterized by relapses. Examples include an elderly woman who begins drinking habitually after the death of her husband; a surgeon who drinks pathologically for a period of time but, when faced with the loss of her practice, receives treatment and recovers; and an individual with a job and family who loses everything due to drinking, becomes homeless for several years, and through involvement with Alcoholics Anonymous (AA), regains his job and family. Some alcoholics never develop serious medical problems, and the majority never seek treatment.

Classifying Alcoholism

There are important aspects of alcohol substance use disorders (SUDs) that should be analyzed. Jellinek was the first to describe subgroups of alcoholism, distinguishing individuals who had persistent alcohol-seeking behaviors and others who could abstain from alcohol for long periods of time, but quickly lost control and could not terminate intake after resumption of drinking (3). More recently, Cloninger et al. described two subtypes of alcoholism (4). Type I alcoholism generally starts with heavy drinking after the age of 25, and intake is reinforced by external circumstances; it includes a greater ability to abstain for long periods of time; and those affected frequently feel loss of control, guilt, and fear about their alcohol dependency. Type II alcoholism includes those who generally have an early onset (before the age of 25) and show spontaneous alcohol-seeking behavior regardless of external circumstances. They have frequent fights and arrests and infrequently experience a feeling of a loss of control, guilt, or fear about alcohol dependency. Interestingly, research on the efficacy of the drug ondansetron in preventing relapse found differences in response between these two groups.

Medical Complications

Adverse physical effects of chronic alcohol abuse include organic mental disorders, diseases of the digestive tract (including liver disease, gastritis, ulcer, pancreatitis, and gastrointestinal cancers), bone marrow suppression, and muscle and hormonal changes. Alcohol has direct toxic effects on the brain, which, combined with metabolic, traumatic, and nutritional deficits, may cause various alcohol-related mental disorders (discussed in Chapter 4, Definition, Presentation, and Diagnosis). Alcohol intake can cause progressive liver damage. Fatty liver develops in nearly anyone with sufficient alcohol intake. Serious alcoholic hepatitis, which can have up to a 50% 5-year mortality rate, may develop. Liver cirrhosis occurs in only approximately 10% of alcoholics; however, 11,000 die from liver disease annually. Of patients with chronic pancreatitis, 75% have an alcohol SUD. Alcohol dissolves mucus and irritates the gastric lining, which contributes to bleeding. Every alcoholic should have a rectal exam with a stool guaiac test as part of a complete physical exam (5).

Alcohol, heavy tobacco use, and deficiencies of vitamins A and B all contribute to high rates of cancer of the mouth, tongue, larynx, esophagus, stomach, liver, and pancreas. Alcoholic patients with oral cancer (to which alcohol significantly contributes) tend to delay onset of treatment longer than most other cancer patients. Early detection is particularly crucial in these diseases. Alcoholic cardiomyopathy can develop after 10 or more years of drinking. Abstinence contributes to recovery in those cases in which damage is not too extensive. Alcohol also has chronic effects on other muscle tissue.

Effects on Blood

Alcoholism is part of the differential diagnosis for anemia, especially megaloblastic anemia. Because of reduced white cell count or further damage to immune functioning, the effects of continued heavy drinking on the possible progression and susceptibility to infection by HIV and progression to AIDS are being studied. For similar reasons, other infectious diseases (e.g., tuberculosis and bacterial pneumonia) have been common among those with alcoholism.

Effects on Hormones

Alcohol interferes with male sexual function and fertility directly through effects on testosterone levels and indirectly through testicular atrophy. Relatively increased levels of estrogen lead to developing gynecomastia and body hair loss. Sexual functioning is affected indirectly through the impact of alcohol on the limbic system and the hypothalamic-pituitary axis. This may be due to vitamin B deficiency or direct toxic effects of alcohol. In women there also may be severe gonadal failure, with an inability to produce adequate quantities of female hormones, affecting secondary sexual characteristics, reducing menstruation, and producing infertility.

Additional Complications

Alcoholism tends to increase blood pressure and is associated with increased risk of cerebrovascular accidents. Alcoholic cerebellar degeneration is a slowly evolving condition encountered along with long-standing histories of excessive use. It affects the cerebellar cortex and produces truncal ataxia and gait disturbances. Alcoholic peripheral neuropathy is characterized by a stocking-and-glove paresthesia, with decreased reflexes and autonomic nerve dysfunction causing, among other problems, impotence. Central pontine myelinolysis is a rare neurological condition of unknown etiology and high mortality. Also of unknown etiology, Marchiafava-Bignami disease is a rare demyelinating disease of the corpus callosum. Computed tomography studies have shown that brain changes that result from alcohol use may be reversible in as little as 3 weeks (6). Alcohol may also impair parasympathetic nerve functioning, which may affect the ability to maintain an erection.

■ SEDATIVES, HYPNOTICS, AND ANXIOLYTICS

The course of CNS depressant abuse/dependence varies from long prodromal periods of use with benzodiazepines or hypnotics, to more rapid onset of addiction with barbiturates, to episodic abuse with other CNS depressants such as methaqualone (Quaalude) or ethchlorvynol (Placidyl). Combinations of CNS depressants with alcohol or with opioids can potentiate the level of intoxication, respiratory depression, and mortality. Chronic sedative abuse can produce blackouts and neuropsychological damage similar to that seen in alcoholism (7). Patients originally using sedatives to treat anxiety will experience an initial anxiety rebound on discontinuation, which in typical abuse is similar to withdrawal in terms of course and symptomatology.

■ OPIOIDS

Intoxication and Withdrawal

Intravenous heroin or opioid intoxication produces a subjective euphoric rush that can be highly reinforcing. Opioid users describe this rush as a feeling of warmth or as an oceanic feeling. The daily use of opioids over days to weeks, depending on the dose and potency of the drug, will produce opioid withdrawal symptoms on cessation of use.

Neonatal Opioid Withdrawal

A syndrome of narcotic abstinence is reported in 60%–94% of neonates of mothers addicted to opioids. Although the baby may appear normal at or shortly after birth, symptoms may appear 12–24 hours later, depending on the half-life of the opioid, and may persist for several months. The full-blown syndrome can include hyperactivity, tremors, seizures, hyperactive reflexes, gastrointestinal dysfunction, respiratory dysfunction, and vague autonomic symptoms (e.g., yawning, sneezing, sweating, nasal congestion, increased lacrimation, and fever). Long-term residual symptoms include infants who appear anxious, hard to please, hyperactive, and emotionally labile.

Adverse Physical Effects

Contaminated needles and impure drugs can lead to endocarditis, septicemia, pulmonary emboli, and pulmonary hypertension. Contaminants can cause skin infections, hepatitis B, and spread of HIV. Death rates in young addicts are increased 20-fold by infection, homicide, suicide, overdose, and (recently) AIDS. Opioid overdose should be suspected in any undiagnosed coma patient, especially along with respiratory depression, pupillary constriction, or presence of needle marks.

Basic research advances in identification of distinct subtypes of opioid receptors have provided increased understanding of the mechanism of cellular opioid neuroregulation and physiology. Cellular mechanisms of opioid receptors are being explored in relation to characteristics of opioid receptors and intracellular modulators of opioid action. Multiple subtypes of opioid receptors designated as mu, delta, kappa, sigma, and epsilon have been described. Neuroadaptation at receptor sites has been hypothesized to produce tolerance and dependence.

Psychosocial Features

Kandel and Faust extensively studied patterns of psychoactive substance abuse in adolescents and young adults and found a progression from tobacco, alcohol, and marijuana to sedatives, cocaine, and opioids (8). Regular marijuana use, development of depressive symptoms, lack of closeness to parents, and dropping out of school may predispose an individual to later narcotic use. Often, opioid abuse is endemic to communities that are economically disadvantaged and have high unemployment, low family stability, and increased tolerance of criminality. These social stressors may result in hopelessness, low self-esteem, poor self-concept, and identification with drug-involved role models and may be intervening variables in the increased opioid dependency rates among minorities. Where poverty and high unemployment are prevalent, many individuals may feel they have little to lose with drug experimentation, and conventional scare tactics have little impact. Alienation from social institutions such as school, increased social deviancy, and impulsivity are high-risk characteristics. There exists a clear association between heroin use and crime. The overwhelming majority of inner-city community members, however, do not use opioids. Research into the factors that are protective for individuals at risk is important.

The Self-Medication Hypothesis

Khantzian found a strong interaction between dominant dysphoric feelings and drug preference (9). The self-medication hypothesis is that the individual self-selects drugs on the basis of personality and ego impairments. Khantzian emphasized an ''antirage property to opioids'' that provides a pharmacological solution or defense against overwhelming anger that is due to either deficient ego defenses or low frustration tolerance. Patients may seek mastery over pain through self-administered drug titration of withdrawal and dysphoria.

Progression

The course of heroin addiction generally involves a 2- to 6-year interval between regular heroin use and seeking of treatment. Early experimentation with opioids may not lead to opioid addiction, but once addiction develops, a lifelong pattern of use and relapse frequently ensues. A preexisting personality disorder may be a factor for drug use progression. The need to secure the drug predisposes the addict to participate in illegal activities or complicates an already existing tendency toward criminality.

■ COCAINE

Natural Course

The majority of casual (especially intranasal) cocaine users do not become dependent, but the widespread thinking in the late 1970s that cocaine was not addictive was mistaken. The time lapse from first use to addiction is usually about 4 years with intranasal use in adults; however, it may be as little as 1.5 years in adolescents. With availability of more potent cocaine derivatives (e.g., crack), experimentation may result in presentation for treatment within months. Most cocaine addicts describe the initial experimentation with cocaine as being fun. At some point in the experience, cocaine use is no longer fun and becomes joyless and compulsive. The activating properties of the drug become more prominent as the euphoria wanes. Cocaine, initially consumed in public places such as bars and at parties, may become an isolating, alienating experience associated with considerable paranoia. A 1-year study in New York City found that in 20% of completed suicides, cocaine had been used immediately prior to suicide (10).

Chronic Use

Chronic cocaine use depletes neurotransmitters and leads to increased receptor sensitivity to dopamine and norepinephrine. These changes are associated with depression, fatigue, poor attention to self-care, poor self-esteem, poor libido, and mild parkinsonism. Tolerance to cocaine does occur, and with continued use, psychosis, an acquired attention-deficit syndrome, and/or stereotypied behaviors become apparent. Given the "fluffy" findings on positron emission tomography scans in such patients, it is assumed that this state is correlated with tissue pathology.

Because of the high cost of cocaine, financial and legal problems may be the first sign of trouble before other stigma of dependence develop. A loss of control, exaggerated involvement, and continued use despite adverse social, occupational, and health effects are criteria pointing to a diagnosis of cocaine dependency.

Adverse Medical Effects

Cocaine has been associated with acute and chronic ailments. Chronic intranasal use has led to nasoseptal defects due to vasoconstriction. Vasodilation also produces nasal stuffiness or "the runs." There is evidence of long-term cerebrovascular disease secondary to long-term cocaine use (11). Anesthetic properties of cocaine may lead to oral numbness and dental neglect. Malnutrition, severe weight loss, and dehydration often result from cocaine binges. Intravenous use of cocaine complicated by impurities may produce endocarditis, septicemia, HIV spread, local vasculitis, hepatitis B, emphysema, pulmonary emboli, and granulomas. Freebase cocaine has been associated with decreased pulmonary exchange, and pulmonary dysfunction may persist. Intravenous cocaine injection sites are characterized by prominent ecchymoses; opioid injection sites more frequently show needle marks.

Positive cocaine urine test results have been increasingly found in homicide victims, in individuals arrested for murder, and in individuals who have died from overdose. Cocaine-induced fatalities have an average blood concentration of 6.2 mg/L (12). Congenital deficiency of pseudocholinesterase may slow down the metabolism and result in toxic levels, sudden delirium, and hypothermia. Deaths in recreational low-dose users have been reported. Acute agitation, diaphoresis, tachycardia, metabolic and respiratory acidosis, cardiac arrhythmia, and grand mal seizures can lead ultimately to respiratory arrest. Recurrent myocardial infarction due to cocaine use associated with tachycardia and coronary vasoconstriction have been reported. Subarachnoid hemorrhage may be precipitated in patients with underlying arterial venous malformations.

Pregnant women who use cocaine may have increased risks for abruptio placenta, and babies who have cocaine-using mothers have been shown to have decreased interactive behavior on Brazelton scales. Further research is being done to study the teratogenicity of cocaine.

■ AMPHETAMINES

Amphetamine abuse may start in conjunction with weight loss treatment, attempts at energy enhancement, or more serious intravenous use. Amphetamine abuse by intravenous administration can present with the same medical complications as seen with intravenous cocaine or heroin use. Amphetamine use shares many similar signs, symptoms, and long-term sequelae with cocaine use.

■ PHENCYCLIDINE/KETAMINE

Chronic psychotic episodes are reported following use of phencyclidine (PCP). With the unpredictability of the experience, it is difficult to explain the abuse of this substance in certain individuals. In contrast to the use of hallucinogens, use of PCP may lead to long-term neuropsychological deficits. PCP abuse may occur in conjunction with multiple substance abuse and may be associated with similar risk factors. Cases of pure PCP abuse have been reported, and in our experience these individuals appear to have significant psychopathology; however, it is difficult to distinguish drug effects from premorbid personality. PCP intoxication produces sympathomimetic- and cholinergic-specific autonomic sequelae and poor function of the cerebellar system including horizontal nystagmus, ataxia, and dizziness.

■ HALLUCINOGENS

Most hallucinogens can produce certain acute adverse effects. The so-called bad trip is a syndrome of anxiety, panic, dysphoria, and paranoia that occurs in the period of intoxication. Because it can lead to suicidal ideation and attempts, the recognition of a bad trip is important. There is no recognized withdrawal syndrome from hallucinogens. Hallucinogen use can also lead to chronic effects including prolonged psychotic states that resemble psychosis or mania. However, syndromes that last longer than 4–6 weeks are generally thought to represent underlying primary psychiatric disease rather than one secondary to these substances. Flashbacks are a different chronic sequela of hallucinogens. Chronic use of hallucinogens has been noted to produce flashback experiences in 15%–30% of chronic users. Prevalence of flashbacks increases with the number of times the individual seeks medical attention, with the exception of flashbacks experienced during acute intoxication or disturbing flashbacks that may be precipitated by other substances such as marijuana. Most strikingly, some hallucinogens have produced permanent parkinsonism by selective destruction of the substantia nigra.

■ CANNABIS

Marijuana abuse tends to begin in adolescence. The use of liquor and cigarettes may be associated with marijuana abuse. Marijuana use has also been described as a precursor to the use of other illegal drugs. It is often used in combinations with other substances (e.g., cocaine). Although many people experiment with marijuana, actual abuse patterns tend to be associated with introduction to drug subcultures among youth, low parental supervision, parental substance abuse, and abuse of drugs by peers. Marijuana abuse should be suspected in someone who has a characteristic set of symptoms, including loss of communication with family, erratic mood changes, deterioration of moral values, apathy, change in friends, truancy, academic underachievement, denial of use even when found having drug paraphernalia, and obvious signs of intoxication.

Adverse Psychological Effects

Generally, the adverse effects of marijuana are not treated in the medical setting. Mild anxiety, depression, and paranoia are frequent occurrences. Several neuropsychological changes and deficits have been identified with marijuana intoxication. Decreases in complex reaction time tasks, digit code memory tasks, fine motor function, time estimation, the ability to track information over time, tactual form discrimination, and concept formation have been found. Such changes translate into impairment in automobile driving, airplane flying, or any other complex motor skill. Difficulties in attention span, coordination, and depth perception have been found up to 10 hours or more after use. Undesirable physical effects include conjunctivitis, dry mouth, and light-headedness. Emotional symptoms of anxiety, confusion, fear, and increased dependency can progress to panic or frank paranoid pathology. Marijuana can also exacerbate depression.

Amotivational Syndrome

A chronic cannabis behavioral syndrome has been called amotivational syndrome (13). This controversial concept describes people who become passive and less goal directed and experience a decrease in motivation, memory, and problem-solving ability after chronic marijuana abuse. Fatigue, apathy, and what has been described as a fog can last for several weeks after cessation of use. Amotivational syndrome has been controversial because of methodological problems in the research. It has been described most frequently in third-world countries, where environmental factors or preexisting personality factors may play a large role.

Adverse Physical Effects

There is increasing evidence that marijuana abuse creates at least some long-term adverse physical effects. For example, several biochemical findings have been reported. Marijuana has been studied in relationship to human male and female fertility, cell metabolism and protein synthesis, normal cell division, and spermatogenesis. Cannabis smoke contains carcinogens similar to tobacco smoke, and chronic marijuana abuse may predispose an individual to chronic obstructive lung disease and pulmonary neoplasm. Cannabis also increases heart rate and blood pressure, which may be crucial in patients with cardiovascular disease. Chronic marijuana abuse may lead to gynecomastia in males. There is some evidence of a marijuana withdrawal syndrome, which should be investigated further.

There are a number of conditions for which marijuana has been suggested as a therapeutic agent. An Institute of Medicine report (14) recommends compassionate use of marijuana products for debilitating medical conditions such as HIV and cancer. Further research is needed in this area.

■ NICOTINE

Course

Tobacco addiction frequently presents as a relapsing condition similar to opioid or cocaine addiction. Cigarette experimentation usually begins in the teenage years. Environmental influences are important; peer tobacco use, parental tobacco use, and use of other substances are contributing factors. Relapse may be evident during periods of high stress, anxiety or maladjustment, poor social support, or low self-confidence. There is a strong association between alcohol and smoking. Frequently, alcoholics are able to stop drinking but have great difficulty giving up smoking at the same time. Many alcohol treatment programs essentially ignore the tobacco addiction; however, tobacco is a major health risk in this population and should be addressed at some point in treatment.

Factors associated with poor long-term outcome consist of poor overall adjustment, poor social support, environmental stress, being around people that continue to smoke, being uninformed about the dangers of cigarette smoking, and having a high level of use or tolerance.

Adverse Medical Sequelae

There are well-known associations between tobacco use and coronary vascular disease, chronic obstructive lung disease, lung cancer, oral cancers, and hypertension. There is growing evidence of its dose-dependent link to cataracts in men. Nicotine tends to increase liver drug metabolism and therefore may lower the levels of medications metabolized by the liver. Psychotropic medications, including neuroleptics and antidepressants, may have lower blood levels in smokers. Smoking is not recommended during pregnancy because smoking is associated with low birth weight.

■ INHALANTS

Course

Inhalant users are predominantly socially economically deprived males 13–15 years of age. Native Americans and teenagers in the Southwest have been found to have a high prevalence of inhalant use. Amyl nitrite use was popular in the 1970s in the homosexual population. Nitrous oxide use may be prevalent among certain health personnel, especially dentists. Most users tend to cease the use after a relatively short period of time and may go on to abuse other psychoactive substances. There is a fairly strong association between aggressive, disruptive, and antisocial behavior and inhalant intoxication.

Adverse Medical Effects

Deaths due to inhalant use have been reported and appear to be caused by central respiratory depression, cardiac arrhythmia, and accidents. Long-term damage to bone marrow, kidneys, liver, neuromuscular tissue, and brain have been reported.

■ REFERENCES

1. Vaillant GE: A long term follow up of male alcohol abuse. Arch Gen Psychiatry 53:243–249, 1996
2. Armor DJ, Polish SM, Stambul HB: Alcoholics and Treatment. New York, Wiley, 1978
3. Jellinek EM: The Disease Concept of Alcoholism. New Haven, CT, Hillhouse Press, 1960
4. Cloninger RC, Sigvardson S, Bohman M: Childhood personality predicts alcohol abuse in young adults. Alcohol Clin Exp Res 12:494–505, 1988
5. Lieber CS: Medical disorders of alcoholism. N Engl J Med 333:1058–1065, 1995
6. Trabert W, Betz T, Niewald M, et al: Significant reversibility of alcoholic brain shrinkage within 3 weeks of abstinence. Acta Psychiatr Scand 92:87–90, 1995
7. Tonne U, Hiltunen AJ, Vilkander B, et al: Neuropsychological changes during steady-state drug use, withdrawal and abstinence in primary benzodiazepine-dependent patients. Acta Psychiatr Scand 91:299–304, 1995
8. Kandel D, Faust R: Sequence and stages in patterns of adolescent drug use. Arch Gen Psychiatry 32:923–932, 1975

9. Khantzian EJ: The self-medication hypothesis of substance use disorders: a reconsideration and recent applications. Harv Rev Psychiatry 4:231–244, 1997

10. Marzuk PM, Tardiff KL, Leon AC, et al: Prevalence of cocaine use among residents of New York City who committed suicide during a one-year period. Am J Psychiatry 149:371–375, 1992

11. Bartzokis G, Beckson M, Hance DB, et al: Magnetic resonance imaging evidence of "silent" cerebrovascular toxicity in cocaine dependence. Biol Psychiatry 45:1203–1211, 1999

12. Spiehler VR, Reed D: Brain concentrations of cocaine and benzoylecgonine in fatal cases. J Forensic Sci 30:1003–1011, 1985

13. Grinspoon L, Bakalar JB: Marihuana, in Substance Abuse: Clinical Problems and Perspectives, 3rd Edition. Edited by Lowinson JL, Ruiz P, Millman RB, Langrod J. Baltimore, MD, Williams and Wilkins, 1997

14. Division of Neuroscience and Behavioral Health, Institute of Medicine: Marijuana and Medicine: Assessing the Science Base. Edited by Joy JE, Watson SJ Jr, Benson JA Jr. Washington, DC, National Academy Press, 1999

8

TREATMENT APPROACHES FOR SUBSTANCE USE DISORDERS

■ ABSTINENCE

The importance of complete abstinence from all substances (except for maintenance replacement and substitution therapies) in the treatment of substance use disorders (SUDs) cannot be overestimated. Partial abstinence, although not ideal, does reduce morbidity and mortality and may be considered an improvement over substance abuse. Nevertheless, although many recovering patients want to continue using alcohol, for example, it is impossible to identify those few for whom controlled drinking is safe. Total abstinence from all substances provides the best prognosis, and all treatment plans should include means to assess for relapse. Dual diagnosis patients need to have antipsychotic and antidepressant medications continued even through relapse.

■ ACHIEVING RECOVERY

The concept of abstinence is different from the concept of recovery or sobriety. Recovery implies the process in which the individual is not only not using drugs, but is also developing a normal, balanced lifestyle, healthy self-esteem, and healthy intimacy in a sense of meaningful living. For addictive patients, recovery is a never-ending process; the term *cure* is avoided.

Relapse Prevention

What is relapse? Is it a return to the preabstinence level of substance use? Is it any substance use at all? Is it a loss of resolution toward changing abuse behavior? Is relapse only the active resuming of substance abuse, or can certain behaviors be labeled on a continuum in the process of relapse? Does the substitution of another form of addictive behavior (e.g., overeating, overworking, or gambling) constitute a relapse?

Relapse is a process of attitudinal change that usually results in use of alcohol or drugs after a period of abstinence. It is an important clinical phenomenon in the course of treating substance abuse. In fact, addiction can be described as a disease with the characteristic of recurrent relapses. More than 90% of patients in any one 12-month period after initiating abstinence will likely use substances; 45%–50% will return to pretreatment levels of substance use (1). Thus it is extremely important that those who have made commitments to recovery understand and anticipate relapse. They need to develop coping strategies and contingency plans to thwart relapse, minimize the extent of damage, and promote renewed abstinence quickly.

Cognitive-behavioral techniques are being used to successfully promote relapse prevention. The patient must understand his or her own unique set of high-risk relapse situations and avoid them or employ coping techniques to avoid relapse when offered substances. Prior to relapse prevention training, a thorough understanding of one's own self-motivational reasons for discontinuing addictive behavior, being able to work through alternative responses to situations, and choosing abstinence as part of the best mode of response is stressed. Marlatt and Gordon identified eight categories of high-risk drinking situations that could be applicable to other substance abuse: unpleasant emotions, physical discomfort, pleasant emotions, testing personal control, urges and temptations, conflict with others, social pressure to drink, and pleasant times with others (2). The one situation providing the highest risk can vary among individuals or drug classes. For example, youths who abuse may be more susceptible to use when experiencing positive feelings. Those who are older and use more chronically may relapse more often because of depression or guilt. Abuse of opiates and cocaine may be more heavily tied to environmental factors. Adolescents may be more susceptible to peer pressure.

It is important to identify and watch for thoughts and feelings that typically occur during high-risk situations. Homework assignments, complete with relapse prevention workbooks, teach patients the ins and outs of the relapse process, help them develop alternative coping skills, and reinforce the experience of a sense of self-mastery in these situations. Relapse prevention is especially valuable in outpatient settings, where opportunities are present to practice skills in a natural environment. Behavioral techniques such as role-playing and assertiveness training are also valuable.

Guilt and Shame Reduction

The clinician expects the patient to see relapse neither as an all-or-none act nor as an unforeseeable or unavoidable event. Relapse, defined as a change in a resolution to change, is a fairly common experience that we all have at times. Relapse, then, is a fact of everyday life. Understanding this may prevent the patient's feeling that he or she has totally failed and that all is lost if a return to use occurs. Marlatt and Gordon coined the term *abstinence violation effect* to describe the view that once use occurs, it must inevitably lead to the pretreatment level of use (2). Guilt, shame, a sense of lack of control, feelings of being trapped, and a lack of a prespecified plan may escalate drug use. The immediate benefit of drug use may overshadow the realization of the negative long-term consequences.

Practicing Social Skills

Identification of personal strengths, past coping behaviors, and environmental supports is important. When faced with temptation or drug use, alternative coping mechanisms include calling a friend or sponsor, leaving the setting, or refusing the next drink. Relapse prevention may require, especially in the early stages of recovery, avoidance of high-risk situations and cues. Later on in the process, some avoidable high-risk situations can be mastered with appropriate coping skills. Social skills training has also been used in prevention. In some situations, however, it may be advisable to avoid cues at all costs (e.g., having a crack addict not return to a setting where cocaine is being used).

Characteristic Predictors of Successful Patient Outcome

Treatment outcome is better in patients with high socioeconomic stability, low antisocial personality, a lack of psychiatric and medical problems, and a negative family history for alcoholism. History of contact with Alcoholics Anonymous (AA), history of a stable job and marriage, and fewer arrests are correlated with a better outcome of treatment. Most studies of treatment settings have not differentiated outcome by treatment setting; however, patients having more medical and psychiatric problems are more often hospitalized and stay longer.

Differential Therapeutics

Despite developments in treatment outcome research, choice of the right treatments for addicted patients is still largely based on the conventional wisdom of clinical considerations. The choice of treatment combinations must be influenced by the fact that many patients have an additional psychiatric illness, multiple addiction is frequent, and selection should fit the unique needs of the patient (3). Other factors to be considered include medical and psychiatric illness, illness severity, characteristics of the individual patient, characteristics of the culture, availability of treatment resources, and awareness of the differential therapeutics of concomitant psychiatric disorders. Recent advances in biobehavioral approaches to psychiatric disorders (i.e., cognitive, behavioral, and psychodynamic individual approaches; and group and family treatment) need to also be considered. Integration of 12-step approaches such as AA, Substance Anonymous, and Narcotics Anonymous (NA) is also highly recommended.

Matching Treatments to Patients

In the past, it was thought that longer inpatient stays were more likely to lead to full or partial abstinence from alcohol and to reduced relapse rates. Today, however, there are more treatment options and more pressure for efficiency. This situation is especially important for patients with SUDs and psychiatric disorders. In a series of classic studies, McLellan et al. (4) found that matching a patient's problems to treatment services improves treatment effectiveness and leads to good overall effectiveness for alcohol treatment. Patients with severe psychiatric problems did poorly regardless of modality or treatment setting. Patients with legal problems did poorly in inpatient programs. Patients with the least severe psychiatric problems did well in inpatient and outpatient settings. Patients with psychiatric problems in the middle range of severity who also had employment or family problems and needed inpatient care improved when psychiatric services were also provided.

■ TREATMENT SETTINGS

Inpatient

Inpatient treatment is indicated for patients with major medical and psychiatric problems and their complications; severe withdrawal symptoms such as delirium tremens (d.t.'s) or seizures; when outpatient treatment, family, friends, or AA members are unable to provide an adequate social support network for abstinence; or in the case of polysubstance addiction. For most other cases, a trial of outpatient treatment is indicated before hospitalization. Patients prefer outpatient treatment, which is less disruptive and more cost-effective than inpatient treatment. Inpatient detoxification is followed by outpatient treatment or by inpatient rehabilitation.

The choice of inpatient rehabilitation in a freestanding substance recovery program, a freestanding inpatient psychiatric hospital, or a general hospital psychiatric unit depends on the severity of additional psychiatric and medical problems. Patients with the most severe psychiatric illness may need to be treated in a locked general hospital inpatient psychiatric unit before transfer to a chemical abuse treatment unit for patients with mental illness.

Treatment outcome is related to treatment length. Patients who complete day hospital substance abuse rehabilitation and then continue to participate in self-help groups are likely to have lower rates of alcohol and cocaine use during follow-up. Furthermore, the beneficial effect of self-help group participation does not appear to be strictly the result of motivation or some other characteristic of the patient.

Outpatient

Outpatient treatment delivery varies from an individual office practitioner, to an addiction day or evening treatment program, to a primary care provider; all may use techniques employed in inpatient treatment programs. Indications for outpatient alcohol detoxification include high motivation and good social support, no previous history of d.t.'s or seizures, brief or not severe recent binges, no severe medical or psychiatric problems or polyaddiction, and prior successful outpatient detoxifications.

■ CLINICAL SITUATIONS

Overdose

More than 5 million poisonings occur each year. Among patients who are alive on arrival to emergency departments (EDs), few die. It can be difficult to empathize with those who repeatedly voluntarily overdose on various drugs. The ED becomes an important evaluation and triage center for these patients.

Treatment of Overdose

Overdose is properly treated in the ED by a medical team. Table 8–1 outlines the major medical complications and treatment approaches to various drug overdoses (5). Because several drugs are slowly absorbed, the minimal time for observation of a suspected drug overdose should be 4 hours. Exact time of ingestion is often difficult to ascertain reliably. If there is good evidence that a specific drug was ingested, a call to the poison control center is suggested, and transfer to an ED is the next step. The first crucial step is to ensure the adequacy of the airway, breathing, and cardiovascular perfusion (ABC), which includes assessment of airway patency, respiratory rate, blood pressure, and pulse. Outside of the hospital, cardiopulmonary resuscitation may be lifesaving. In the medical setting, an individual who has overdosed and is unconscious or any individual whose etiology of coma is unknown should receive 50 mg of dextrose (5% in water) and 0.4 mg of naloxone, which may need to be repeated. Prompt response supports evidence for hypoglycemia, opiate overdose, or alcohol overdose. In the case of Wernicke's encephalopathy, dextrose should not be given first because glucose can further suppress thiamine stores. Other basic measures include diazepam treatment for status epilepticus and treatment of metabolic acidosis.

Elimination Methods

We emphasize general parameters (Table 8–2) for elimination; for technical information on elimination, refer to Goldberg et al. (6). Gastric emptying is appropriate only for drugs orally ingested. One absolute contraindication to gastric emptying is in cases of caustic ingestion. Ipecac syrup induces vomiting in approximately 30 minutes; to reduce the risk of aspiration it should be given only to patients who are awake and alert. It should be given even after spontaneous emesis because full gastric emptying may not have been accomplished. Gastric lavage entails flushing the upper gastrointestinal system with water. This technique is attempted only with patients who are unconscious and whose airway is secured by intubation. Placed in the stomach, activated charcoal serves as an absorbent to remove toxic substances, and it may reduce reabsorption of substances from the duodenum. When ingested substances

TABLE 8-1. **Management of overdose**

Drug	Major complications	Antidote/treatment	Potential lethal dose
Acetaminophen	Hepatotoxicity: peaks at 72–96 hours. Complete recovery generally in 4 days, but injury worse for alcoholics. Mortality: 1%–2%.	Acetylcysteine	140 mg/kg
Alcohol	Respiratory depression	None	350–700 mg (serum)
Amphetamines	Seizures; avoid neuroleptics	None	20–25 mg/kg
Short-acting barbiturate	Respiratory depression	None	>3 g
Long-acting barbiturate	Respiratory depression	None	>6 g
Benzodiazepine	Sedation, respiratory depression, hypotension, coma	Flumazenil reverses effects (but it may induce withdrawal in the dependent)	
Carbon monoxide	Headaches, dizziness, weakness, nausea, vomiting, diminished visual acuity, tachycardia, tachypnea, ataxia, and seizures are all possible. Other manifestations include hemorrhages (cherry red spots on the skin), metabolic acidosis, coma, and death.	Hyperbaric oxygen	

Cocaine	Peak toxicity 60–90 minutes after use; systemic sympathomimesis and seizures, acidosis. Later cardiopulmonary depression, perhaps pulmonary edema. Treatment of acidosis, seizures, and hypertension is imperative.	Narcan (empirically)	Varies with tolerance
Nonbenzodiazepine hypnotics	Delirium, extrapyramidal syndrome	None	
Hydrocarbons	Gastrointestinal, repiratory, and CNS compromise	None	
Opioids	Miosis, respiratory depression, obtundation, pulmonary edema, delirium, death	Naloxone, nalmefene helpful	Varies with tolerance
Phencyclidine/ ketamine	Hypertension, nystagmus, rhabdomyolysis	None. Forced diuresis should not be attempted in cases of PCP overdose with suspected rhabdomyolysis.	
Phenothiazines	Anticholinergism, extrapyramidal side effects, cardiac effects	Phenothiazine overdose should be monitored for 48 hours for cardiac arrhythmia. Lidocaine may be necessary for treatment of cardiac arrhythmia, norepinephrine for hypotension, sodium bicarbonate for metabolic acidosis, and Dilantin for seizures.	150 mg/kg

TABLE 8–1. **Management of overdose** (*continued*)

Drug	Major complications	Antidote/treatment	Potential lethal dose
Salicylates	CNS, acidosis	None	500 mg/kg
Tricyclics	Cardiac effects, hypotension, anticholinergism	None	35 mg/kg
Hallucinogens	Ring-substituted amphetamines, even LSD/mescaline may lead to rhabdomyolysis, hyperthermia, hyponatremia	Reduce temperature, administer dantrolene	
Inhalants	Cardiotoxicity, arrhythmias	Cardiac monitoring	

Note. See Chapter 4, Definition, Presentation, and Diagnosis, for further descriptions of overdose states.

TABLE 8–2. Overdose elimination methods

Drug	Ipecac syrup	Forced diuresis	Gastric lavage	Activated charcoal	Hemodialysis	Hemoperfusion
Acetaminophen	Yes	Yes (alkaline)	Yes	No	No	No
Alcohol	No	No	Yes	Yes	Yes	No
Amphetamines	Yes	Yes (acid)	Yes	Yes	Yes	NA
Barbiturates	NA	Only for long-acting	NA	Yes	NA	Yes
Benzodiazepines	Yes	No	Yes	Repeated	NA	NA
Carbon monoxide	No	No	No	No	No	No
Cocaine	No	No	No	No	No	No
Nonbenzodiazepine hypnotics	Yes	No	Yes	Yes	NA	NA
Hydrocarbons	Yes	NA	Yes (if orally ingested)	NA	NA	NA
Opioids	NA	NA		NA	NA	NA
Phencyclidine/ketamine	Only severe	Not in rhabdomyolysis (avoid in renal failure)	Only severe	Yes	NA	NA
Phenothiazines	Yes	NA	Yes	Yes	NA	NA
Salicylates	Yes	Yes (alkaline)	Yes	Yes	Yes	NA
Tricyclics	NA	NA	NA	Repeated	No	No

Note. This table covers elimination of substances and does not necessarily include "antidotes" or medications that are covered in Table 8–1. "No" refers to a specific contraindication of that particular method in overdose of that substance. "NA" implies that the method has not been studied or is not applicable to overdose of that substance.

are weak acids or bases, forced diuresis can be attempted in patients with functioning kidneys. Dialysis is generally a heroic measure to save a life and is most successful for drugs that are circulating in the plasma, minimally bound to tissue, and cleared poorly through the kidney. Dialysis has been especially valuable in cases of alcohol, amphetamine, and aspirin overdose. Hypoperfusion is an extracorporeal blood-filtering technique similar to dialysis that uses a different type of membrane filtration. Hypoperfusion has been especially useful in barbiturate overdose; however, it may lead to thrombocytopenia.

■ INTOXICATION

Most simple intoxication does not come to medical attention. Those cases that do present to the ED should be screened carefully for medical problems such as subdural hematomas, meningitis, HIV infection, or endocarditis with embolization. Support measures include interrupting substance absorption, providing a safe environment, decreasing sensory stimulation, and allowing the passage of time. A calm, nonthreatening manner should be employed, with clear communication and reality orientation. Attempts to reason with most intoxicated patients will not be fruitful; in cases of hallucinogen abuse, however, individuals can frequently be talked down from pathological intoxication.

Alcohol

There is no proven amethystic agent that can hasten the cessation of alcohol intoxication (not even strong black coffee or cold showers). Experimental approaches to delaying absorption or decreasing metabolism and elimination have been numerous, and opiate antagonists (including naloxone) and CNS stimulants have also been studied as means to protect against dangerous effects of intoxication. The safe passage of time is currently the only effective measure to reverse acute intoxication.

Opioids

No specific measures are generally needed to treat opioid intoxication. If life-threatening overdose is suspected, prompt treatment with naloxone is necessary (see above and Table 8–1).

Cocaine and Amphetamines

Cocaine abusers often self-medicate with CNS depressants to antagonize the dysphoric stimulant properties of the drug. For severe agitation, benzodiazepines such as diazepam and lorazepam may be helpful. If frank psychosis persists, low-dose haloperidol (2–5 mg) may be helpful, and the dose should be adjusted as necessary to control symptoms. However, haloperidol will also decrease the seizure threshold and should be used with caution. Monoamine oxidase inhibitors (MAOIs) should be avoided because they inhibit the degradation of cocaine and can produce a hypertensive crisis.

PCP

The fundamental goal in treating the violence associated with PCP intoxication is to ensure the safety of all parties. When a patient becomes threatening, the strong physical presence of at least five people is needed for physical containment. Benzodiazepines, such as diazepam, are superior to neuroleptics during treatment of agitation, but neuroleptics such as haloperidol are better for PCP toxic psychosis. Enhancement of excretion is helpful, with gastric lavage if orally administered or by acidification of the urine if systemic. For lasting problems, electroconvulsive therapy may be indicated.

Cannabis

Cannabis intoxication generally needs no formal treatment. The occasional severe anxiety attacks or acute paranoid episodes can be handled by reality orientation. Severe anxiety may rarely warrant treatment with a benzodiazepine, and low-dose haloperidol or olanzapine may be helpful for cannabis psychosis.

Hallucinogens

Patients experiencing hallucinogen intoxication can be talked down with reality orientation and reassurance. Benzodiazepines may help to provide sedation. Overdose, especially of ecstasy, can lead to hyperpyrexia, dehydration, tachycardia, and even death and should be treated in a medical setting.

Inhalants

Inhalant intoxication can vary in its presentation and need for active treatment. The main principle is protection of the individual from harm and from harming others. Symptoms are usually time limited.

■ ALCOHOL WITHDRAWAL

Inpatient Versus Outpatient Setting

For treatment of alcohol SUDs, patients with delirium, low IQ, Wernicke's encephalopathy, trauma history, neurological symptoms, medical complications, psychopathology that requires medication, d.t.'s, or alcoholic seizures or hallucinosis are probably best evaluated and treated in an inpatient setting (Table 8–3). Polysubstance abuse, poor compliance, poor family support, lack of trans-

TABLE 8–3.	Medical workup for alcohol withdrawal
Routine lab tests	CBC with differential, serum electrolytes, liver function tests including bilirubin, BUN, and creatinine levels, fasting blood sugar, prothrombin time, cholesterol level, triglyceride level, calcium, magnesium, albumin, total protein, hepatitis B surface antigen, B_{12}, folate, stool guaiac, urinalysis, serum and urine toxic screens, chest X ray, ECG
Ancillary tests	Electroencephalogram, computed tomography, gastrointestinal series, HIV, VDRL

portation, a chaotic or unstable home environment, or an environment in which the patient is continually exposed to others with SUDs all predict poor outpatient detoxification success. Yet, outpatient detoxification can be appropriate: approximately 95% of patients have only mild to moderate withdrawal symptoms. Supportive care without pharmacological intervention is adequate for a significant number of these patients, and even when pharmacological treatment is needed, it can be given in an outpatient setting. Outpatient care reduces costs, allows the patient to continue to function in his or her environment, and provides time for the therapist to evaluate the patient's motivation for treatment.

Pharmacological Versus Nonpharmacological Treatment

Most withdrawing alcohol users do not have major medical problems; still, the best treatment approach is conservative psychopharmacological management. Use of medication for the prevention of d.t.'s or seizures is a top priority not only to avoid discomfort and death, but also to avoid the acceleration of cognitive decline secondary to repeated uncontrolled withdrawal. Thus pharmacological detoxification is warranted for those with significant signs of withdrawal, codependence on other CNS depressants, a clear history of severe daily dependence or high tolerance, or a history of d.t.'s or seizures. Medical complications (e.g., infections, trauma, metabolic or hepatic disorders) indicate pharmacological treatment. Physical and subjective discomfort should be minimized. Pharmacological care enhances compliance and provides an alcohol-free interval that may help the patient commit to treatment. Negative countertransference of staff members can result in withholding of appropriate medication. There should be little to no concern that this treatment will make the alcoholic patient abuse benzodiazepines.

Nonpharmacological detoxification is for patients with mild symptoms or withdrawal history and mild-to-moderate dependence. Patients are housed for 3–4 days in a supportive, safe environment with rest and nutrition and detoxified without medication. This helps the patient to regulate and structure his or her life again. Close monitoring of patients for complications and adequate medical backup is needed for detoxification.

Pharmacological Withdrawal

All patients withdrawing from alcohol should be carefully monitored for vital signs, physical signs, and subjective symptoms at least every 4 hours while awake (Table 8–3). Several objective rating scales and some subjective scales (e.g., the Clinical Institute Withdrawal Assessment [7] for those without general medical complications) are used to monitor the withdrawal state. In pharmacological detoxification, a substitute drug that is cross-tolerant with alcohol is administered and slowly withdrawn from the body. For withdrawing patients with an altered mental status due to conditions other than alcohol (e.g., other substances, general medical or surgical conditions), detoxification remains a priority. Indeed, for those withdrawing from both opioids and alcohol, benzodiazepines might be given preferentially to methadone in order to substitute the alcohol while avoiding excessive sedation.

Benzodiazepine Treatment

Many agents somewhat benefit the withdrawal state, but with their agonist effect at the gamma-aminobutyric acid (GABA) receptor, benzodiazepines are currently the best medications for alcohol detoxification. With adequate benzodiazepine coverage, complications of alcohol withdrawal are extremely rare. At usual doses, benzodiazepines produce little respiratory depression and have a good margin of safety between effective dose and overdose. Chlordiazepoxide (Librium) and diazepam (Valium), the most commonly used benzodiazepines, are long acting. Once a sufficient dose has been given, they can be expected to self-taper without further dosing needed. With a lesser risk of accumulation and overdose, intermediate half-life benzodiazepines such as lorazepam (Ativan) and oxazepam (Serax) are useful in patients with hepatic disease, delirium, dementia, or pulmonary disease, or with elderly patients. Lorazepam also has the advantages of primarily renal clearance and reliable intramuscular absorption. Table 8–4 shows treatment protocols for withdrawal. In all cases, thiamine (100 mg) administered orally or intramuscularly, folic acid (1–3 mg), and multivitamins should also be added. When indicated, naltrexone or disulfiram (Antabuse) can be added after completion of a physical examination, an electrocardiogram, and blood work, in the absence of contraindications such as arrhythmias, heart disease, severe hepatic disease, esophageal varices, pregnancy, or epilepsy (discussed below), and after at least 72 hours since last ingestion of alcohol.

Suppression of withdrawal symptoms does not substitute for systematic detoxification. A conservative 5- to 7-day regimen (Table 8–4) promotes comfort, reduces complications, provides structure, and helps most patients cope cognitively and emotionally with the initial treatment. Uncomplicated detoxification of this length rarely occurs in an inpatient unit because of cost pressures, and inpatient alcohol detoxification is often condensed to 3 days. Out-

---

TABLE 8–4. **Benzodiazepine treatment for alcohol withdrawal**

Outpatient	Chlordiazepoxide 25–50 mg po qid on first day, 20% decrease over 5 days, daily visits.
Inpatient	1. Choose agent: diazepam or chlordiazepoxide. Give initial loading dose then monitor objectively every 2–4 hours using vital signs, the Clinical Institute Withdrawal Assessment (CIWA) scale, or both.
	2. Give additional dose every 2–4 hours as needed: chlordiazepoxide 25–50 mg (maximum 400 mg/24 hours), diazepam 5–10 mg (maximum 100 mg/24 hours), oxazepam 15–30 mg, or lorazepam 1 mg.
	3. Count total dose needed for stabilization of signs.
	4. Total divided by 4 is amount to give four times a day.
	5. Taper daily total about 25% over 3 days; continue no more than 10 days.
	6. Use adjunctive treatments.
	7. Thiamine 100 mg, 4 times a day; folate 1 mg, 4 times a day; multivitamin each day; $MgSO_4$ 1 g im every 6 hours for 2 days if seizures occur (or carbamazepine or valproate).

patient detoxification for uncomplicated alcohol dependence can be accomplished with chlordiazepine (25 mg qid) decreasing to zero within 4–5 days. Inpatient withdrawal from alcohol is accomplished with chlordiazepoxide (Librium) orally (25–100 mg qid with 25–50 mg every 2 hours prn) for positive withdrawal signs. Doses can be held if the patient appears intoxicated. Both regimens should include thiamine (50–100 mg) orally or intramuscularly, multivitamins, and folate (1–3 mg/day). Naltrexone is usually added 5 days after detoxification.

Adjuncts to Benzodiazepines

Seizure Protection

Consideration of patients at imminent risk of withdrawal seizures or d.t.'s should be a part of all detoxification strategies. Physicians do not regularly prescribe antiepileptic drugs prophylactically unless the patient has a history of a seizure disorder. Those who have had seizures during withdrawal do not regularly take anticonvulsant medications. Gabapentin, which lacks significant drug-to-drug interactions, cognitive effects, and abuse potential, is an ideal medication for patients who have had seizures during withdrawal. Phenytoin was previously used for these patients, and valproate may be used as well. Magnesium sulfate (1 g qid for 2 days) is also useful.

Autonomic Signs

Both beta-blockers (e.g., propranolol) and alpha-blockers (e.g., clonidine) may alleviate autonomic nervous system signs and symptoms that occur during withdrawal. A usual dose of propranolol is 10 mg every 6 hours as needed, and a usual dose for clonidine is 0.5 mg 2–3 times a day as needed.

Psychotic Features

Neuroleptics are helpful for delirium, delusions, or hallucinations. Haloperidol (0.5–2.0 mg) can be administered intramuscularly every 2 hours.

Other CNS Depressants

Withdrawal from benzodiazepines, barbiturates, or other depressants often requires pharmacological detoxification. This is true for benzodiazepines used in high doses for short periods or low to medium dosages for long periods (i.e., months, years). Conservative treatment requires a slow withdrawal over many days or weeks. Withdrawal from benzodiazepines generally can be performed with chlordiazepoxide or diazepam (long half-life). A standard benzodiazepine detoxification regimen is outlined in Table 8–5. If the abuse history is unreliable or difficult to ascertain, a pentobarbital challenge test can be used to find a starting dose (Table 8–6). Benzodiazepine detoxification is best done in an inpatient unit except for those who have been on a low dose for a very long time. Outpatient detoxification for those who have used benzodiazepines chronically at low doses occurs over 6–12 weeks of gradual reduction, wherein added support and education are helpful. The option of an as-needed dose to avoid feeling trapped is fine. The worst symptoms occur at the lowest doses and in the first week without any medication. All parties should be prepared: the stress of that week may seem to last a year.

After detoxification, patients should be referred to AA or NA and Al-Anon. For those who originally presented with anxiety, rebound can be expected. Nonbenzodiazepine alternatives for anxiety might include cognitive-behavioral therapy (CBT), exercise, relax-

---

TABLE 8–5. **Benzodiazepine detoxification**

1. Establish usual maintenance dose by history or pentobarbital tolerance test (Table 8–6).
2. Divide maintenance dose into equivalent as-needed doses of diazepam and administer first 2 days.
3. Decrease diazepam 10% each day thereafter.
4. Administer diazepam 5 mg every 6 hours as needed for signs of increased withdrawal.
5. When diazepam dose approaches 10% of original, reduce dose slowly over 3–4 days, then discontinue.

TABLE 8–6. **Pentobarbital challenge test**

Patient condition after test dose	Degree of tolerance	Estimated 24-hour pentobarbital requirement (mg)
Asleep, but arousable	None or minimal	None
Drowsy; slurred speech; ataxia; marked intoxication	Definite but mild	400–600
Comfortable; fine lateral nystagmus only	Marked	600–1000
No signs of effect; abstinence signs persist	Extreme	1000–1200 or more; in this case give 100 mg every 2 hours until mild intoxication is produced (to a maximum of 500 mg). Multiply the amount that produced mild intoxication by 4, which is the estimated 24-hour dose of pentobarbital, and convert to phenobarbital equivalents (30 mg of phenobarbital equals 100 mg of pentobarbital). Give that phenobarbital dose for 2 days and then taper by 30 mg/day or 10% per day.

Note. For benzodiazepine discontinuation: see clinical response 1 hour after 200-mg test dose of pentobarbital.

ation, or psychotherapy. One in eight patients who go through detoxification will develop severe anxiety that requires treatment with medications and/or CBT.

Many CNS depressants such as glutethimide (Doriden) are abused episodically and do not require formal detoxification. For barbiturate or methaqualone abuse, detoxification is necessary. Barbiturates can be detoxified with a long-acting benzodiazepine or a long-acting barbiturate, such as phenobarbital.

In some cases there is a need to substitute one CNS depressant for another. Most such cross-tapers occur over 3 weeks using clonazepam. In week 1, use clonazepam (0.5 mg) at bedtime and the previously used drug as required. In week 2, discontinue the previously used drug. In week 3, reduce the clonazepam to zero. This regimen requires inpatient admission in cases of nonbenzodiazepine treatment, polysubstance abuse, or outpatient failures. The pentobarbital tolerance test should be used to set the initial dose when dosage of use is unknown. Alprazolam (Xanax) is uniquely less amenable to drug substitution. Breakthrough seizures have been reported despite adequate coverage with chlordiazepoxide. Alprazolam detoxification should include an estimation of daily use and a slow withdrawal over a period of several weeks. Clonazepam has also been successfully used in alprazolam detoxification.

■ OPIOIDS

Opioid Detoxification

Opioid detoxification may be necessary to interrupt an opioid-related SUD. Individuals with opioid-related SUDs rarely seek treatment, but when they do, circumstances may coincide with an interrupted supply of the substance, an overdose, or an attempt at self-detoxification. Methadone detoxification can be difficult because of methadone's long half-life and usual chronic use. The most common approach to opioid detoxification is to substitute methadone for the opioid that has been used and then to gradually decrease the methadone dose. For most heroin addicts, 20 mg of methadone is adequate, and the patient should be reevaluated every 2–4 hours in case additional dosage is necessary. Once a stable dose is achieved, methadone should be decreased by, usually, 5 mg/day over a period of 4–14 days. When deciding on an initial dose, note that pure drug to methadone ratios are as follows: heroin to methadone, 2:1; morphine sulfate to methadone; 4:1; meperidine to methadone, 20:1; codeine to methadone, 50:1; and oxycodone to methadone, 12:1.

Another approach to opioid detoxification is to administer the abused drug and slowly taper its dose over time. Although this approach is untenable for illicit drugs, codeine, for example, can be detoxified in this way. The estimated amount used daily is mixed with 30 mg of cherry syrup and given every day for 7–10 days, and the amount of drug is decreased daily. A low dose (25–50 mg) of thioridazine (Mellaril) concentrate can be added to reduce subjective discomfort.

Clonidine is an alpha-2 agonist (see below) that effectively suppresses signs and symptoms of autonomic sympathetic activation during withdrawal (it has been less successful in decreasing the subjective discomfort of withdrawal). Clonidine detoxification is most successful for individuals with mild dependence and high motivation, and who have inpatient status. On the first day of treatment, clonidine is administered orally in a range of 0.1–0.3 mg tid (max 1.2 mg) and increased on the third day to 0.4–0.7 mg tid for a total detoxification period of 10–14 days. In appropriate patients, naltrexone treatment can be started during the clonidine detoxification as described in Table 8–7 (8). The major side effects of clonidine administration are hypotension and sedation. Vital signs should be monitored carefully for patients taking clonidine. Highly motivated patients can undergo clonidine detoxification in an outpatient setting (9). Lofexidine, a centrally acting alpha-2 agonist, may be comparable to clonidine but is not yet approved by the U.S. Food and Drug Administration (FDA) for this purpose.

Rapid and ultrarapid detoxification approaches use opioid antagonists and adjuncts such as clonidine detoxification, sedation, and even general anesthesia and are performed at few institutions. These approaches are used for those in transition to antagonist ther-

TABLE 8–7. Ambulatory opioid detoxification medication protocols

Nine-day clonidine detoxification

Nine-day protocol	Day 1	Days 2, 3, 4	Days 5, 6, 7	Days 8, 9
Clonidine	0.1–0.2 mg; max dose: 1 mg	0.1–0.2 mg po qid prn; max dose: 1.4 mg	Taper to zero	Zero
Naltrexone				Day 8: 25 mg, day 9: 50 mg

Five-day detoxification with clonidine ending with induction of naltrexone 50 mg/day

Five-day protocol	Days 1, 2	Days 3, 4, 5
Clonidine	Preload: 0.2–0.4 mg tid; max dose: 1.2 mg	Taper to zero
Oxazepam	Preload 30–60 mg	Zero
Naltrexone	Day 1: 12.5 mg, day 2: 25 mg	50 mg po each day

apy. Unfortunately, ultrarapid detoxification has the increased risks of anesthesia, is done without rehabilitation, and is expensive.

Detoxification Adjuncts

Detoxification using clonidine as an adjunct should take 5–6 days; it is unlikely to help beyond 14 days. It can be administered transdermally using a patch. Clonidine should be avoided at night. Benzodiazepines are helpful for insomnia. At low doses, buprenorphine is useful as a partial agonist because it blocks withdrawal (2–4 mg per day), but at larger doses it decreases respiratory drive. Other drugs that help to alleviate discomfort during withdrawal include dicyclomine (Bentyl) for gastrointestinal pain, nonsteroidal anti-inflammatory drugs for myalgias, and antiemetics.

Maintenance Treatment

Maintenance treatment is provided by substitution of an opioid agonist. The standard agonist used in substitution is methadone, but new agents such as buprenorphine and L-alpha acetyl methadol (LAAM) are also effective in the attempt to interrupt the addictive lifestyle, promote stability and employment, reduce intravenous drug use and hence the risk of hepatitis B or HIV infection, and reduce criminal activity. Methadone is a long-acting (half-life 24–36 hours), cross-tolerant opioid that mutes extreme fluctuation in serum opioid level and blunts euphoric response to heroin. Given once daily, it provides a structure for rehabilitation. Starting doses are usually 20–40 mg, depending on degree of dependence, and may require an increase to 120 mg/day. Maintenance at doses of 70 mg and above leads to fewer relapses. NA-oriented rehabilitations or therapeutic communities may exclude patients who take methadone. Debate surrounds the substitution model, but the positive effects of methadone are vital to a subset of patients.

A large number of patients have successfully interrupted their drug lifestyle using methadone maintenance. Unfortunately, only 20%–25% of those who are addicted get this treatment. It is primarily indicated for the patient with hard-core addiction and for patients who are HIV positive, pregnant, or who have a history of legal problems. Methadone maintenance is contraindicated for anyone who is younger than age 16, who is to be jailed within 30–45 days, or who has a history of abusing the medicine. Many addicted patients have compromised liver function due to alcohol abuse or hepatitis, and methadone use may be contraindicated with severe liver damage. Many individuals take methadone for several years. When indicated, it should be withdrawn slowly to minimize discomfort; methadone withdrawal is often a protracted affair. Generally the medication should not be decreased more than 10% per week. Below 10–20 mg of methadone, subjective symptoms of withdrawal may intensify and necessitate a further decrease in the rate of withdrawal to 3% per week.

LAAM, a long-acting methadone derivative, is another long-acting mu agonist, and its use in maintenance treatment is similar to that of methadone. LAAM and its metabolites have a longer half-life than does methadone and need less frequent dosing. A 60- to 100-mg dose of LAAM taken three times weekly is equivalent to a 50- to 100-mg dose of methadone taken daily.

Buprenorphine (Buprenex) is a mixed agonist-antagonist that has lower addictive properties, fewer withdrawal symptoms, and a lower overdose risk (because of its antagonist properties). Its efficacy in reducing illicit opioid use has been documented (10). Buprenorphine and low-dose methadone (20–30 mg) are comparable in terms of efficacy of program retention and illicit use.

Iatrogenic withdrawal often leads to relapse. Frequent detoxifications with methadone with subsequent relapses can be avoided by methadone maintenance. It is useful to remember the half-lives of the opioids: morphine sulfate, 2–3 hours; methadone, 15–25 hours; and LAAM, 55 hours. LAAM needs to be given only three times per week, and on cessation there should be no withdrawal for 72–96 hours.

Antagonist Maintenance

Naltrexone is an opioid antagonist (see below) that when used regularly leads to gradual extinction of drug-seeking behavior. For opioid relapse prevention, naltrexone is usually given in a dose of

25–50 mg/day over the initial 5–10 days and gradually increased to 50–100 mg daily or three times weekly. High refusal and drop-out rates limit its use to highly motivated individuals with a good prognosis who are likely to do well in a variety of treatment options and with whom there is a good treatment alliance. Naltrexone can be used in the outpatient setting over the long term. It is valuable in abstinence-oriented treatment. Naltrexone may induce withdrawal when given to someone who has used opioids within the previous 7 days; the clinician should determine the risk of this situation.

■ COCAINE, CANNABIS, HALLUCINOGENS, AND INHALANTS

There are no specific pharmacological detoxification procedures for cocaine, cannabis, hallucinogens, and inhalants. General support measures are usually adequate. Acupuncture may be an aid to cocaine detoxification. Benzodiazepines may help the patient withdrawing from cocaine, but they have the potential for abuse. Other medications that may help alleviate the symptoms of cocaine abstinence include desipramine (which is superior to lithium), carbamazepine and other antidepressants, and perhaps buprenorphine when opioids have been used in addition to cocaine. Suicide precautions should be taken with such patients when they are depressed or psychotic.

For inhalant-induced psychosis, the efficacy of carbamazepine compares to that of haloperidol but without the extrapyramidal side effects or lowering of seizure threshold (11).

The dangerous amphetamine-like state caused by ring-substituted amphetamine hallucinogens (MDMA, MDA) should be closely monitored; supportive treatment, including hydration and monitoring for hyperpyrexia and perhaps dantrolene, should be provided as needed. The sympathomimetic state produced by LSD and mescaline also requires support. Patients experiencing anxiety due to use of LSD and mescaline need reassurance and reorientation. Usually restraint can be avoided. For the psychological sequelae of hallucinogens, benzodiazepines are superior to typical neuroleptics.

■ NICOTINE

A number of guidelines for smoking cessation have been established (12). Relapse, unfortunately, is the rule within 3 months. The primary care provider's assistance is essential. Compliance with the nicotine patch is greater than with nicotine chewing gum. Bupropion in the sustained release form (Zyban) is helpful. Scheduled dosing may be better than dosing as required. A nasal spray is also available but is not superior. Neither fluoxetine nor clonidine is helpful.

■ POLYSUBSTANCE ABUSE

Detoxification

Polysubstance abuse makes detoxification more difficult. Concurrent withdrawal from multiple substances confuses the clinical picture. For detoxification from both CNS depressants and opioids, detoxification of the former is the priority because of the life-threatening nature of CNS depressant withdrawal and the length of opiate detoxification. Also, combining benzodiazepines and methadone risks the possibility of overdose and requires close patient monitoring and dose adjustments as needed. Simultaneous detoxification from different classes of drugs can greatly increase physical or psychological discomfort and lead to higher elopement or relapse.

Integration of Treatment Approaches

Polysubstance abuse has been inadequately addressed by the treatment system. Drug and alcohol programs are often separately funded. Alcohol counselors may lack the training or interest to treat polysubstance abuse. Until recently, AA groups had difficulty integrating younger polysubstance abusers into their membership. Unfortunately, an attitude that one addiction is more important than another can develop. In clinical settings, such attitudes must be confronted with education and greater tolerance of social differences among patients. The exclusively alcoholic middle-aged white male, once common in treatment facilities, is now outnumbered by a younger, polyaddicted, and more heterogeneous population with additional psychiatric problems.

■ TREATMENT MODALITIES

Psychosocial Treatments

Treatment is not simply counseling. Dialectical behavioral therapy (DBT), interpersonal psychotherapy (IPT), CBT, motivational interviewing, and psychodynamically oriented psychotherapy are important treatment modalities, although their benefit is often delayed. Data show that psychotherapy combined with certain psychopharmacological treatments is more efficacious than either treatment alone (13). There are some cases in which the medication is absolutely needed.

Individual Therapy

Individual therapy can be conducted alone or with other modalities, including pharmacotherapy, 12-step programs, and family and group treatments. Abstinence is an important measure of efficacy and should be considered as a goal and a means to treatment success. Treatments range from psychodynamically informed supportive and expressive treatment to cognitive, behaviorally oriented treatment. Individual treatments are especially indicated when patients face bereavement, loss, or social disruption and have targeted problems (e.g., anxiety disorders or panic disorders). Brief interventions are sometimes effective and worth an attempt, especially in primary care settings; however, many patients require long-term care and follow-up.

Initiating Individual Treatment: The Therapeutic Contract

At the outset, the therapist should concentrate on how the patient can accept his or her problem and on the treatment necessary for the patient to achieve and maintain sobriety. The contract between the patient and the therapist should address treatment frequency and modality, a limit to the continuation of treatment despite continued use, inclusion of significant others in the social network, a clear goal of abstinence, psychopharmacological treatment if indicated, and arrangements regarding cost and time of treatment.

The Individual Psychotherapies

Psychodynamically Oriented Therapy

Psychodynamically oriented individual treatment is for patients with problems in identity, separation and individuation, affect regulation, self-governance, and self-care. For those with addictive disorders and other neurotic problems, psychodynamically oriented therapy requires psychological mindedness; capacity for honesty, intimacy, and identification with the therapist; average to superior intelligence; economic stability; high motivation; and a willingness to discuss conflict. Expressive psychotherapy may lead to deepening of a capacity to tolerate depression and anxiety without substance use. When patients are not abstinent, exploratory treatment may do more harm than good, with reactivation of painful conflicts leading to further drinking and regression (14). Formal psychoanalysis is contraindicated in early phases of addictive treatment, especially in patients who are actively drinking. If abstinent, however, some patients respond well to insight-oriented psychotherapy.

Cognitive-Behavioral Therapy

Cognitive-behavioral therapy (CBT) has been modified for SUDs (15). The assumption of CBT is that abuse and dependence on substances are learned behaviors and can be changed. CBT is a treatment in which the patient works to identify and modify maladaptive thought patterns that lead to feelings that lead to use. It is very helpful for relapse prevention and for patients who are dependent, sociopathic, or who have primary psychiatric symptoms. CBT has been helpful for prevention of relapse to cocaine use.

Dialectical Behavioral Therapy

Dialectical behavioral therapy (DBT) is a comprehensive, behaviorally oriented treatment designed for highly dysfunctional patients meeting criteria for borderline personality disorder. Many of these criteria are characteristic of drug abusers and some of the problems encountered in treatment of drug abusers, especially when various treatments are combined. The basic challenge of the DBT therapist is the balancing of validation and acceptance treatment strategies with problem-solving procedures, including contingency management, exposure-based procedures, cognitive modification, and skills training. DBT has been shown to be more effective than other treatments in treating drug abuse in women with borderline personality disorder (16).

Motivational Enhancement Therapy

Motivational enhancement therapy is a directive, empathic patient-centered counseling style that addresses the patient's ambivalence and denial. Ideally, motivational enhancement therapy will motivate the patient and make brief interventions more effective by taking the patient through stages of denial and cooperation. At the right stage of recovery, the contribution of primary care motivational intervention is potentially great and should be pursued by generalists (17, 18).

Group Therapy

Group therapy is frequently the principal treatment modality for addictive disorders. Groups provide opportunities for resocialization and opportunities to practice social skills, object relatedness, and impulse control; they foster one's identity as a recovering person and support acceptance of abstinence. They raise patients' self-esteem and support reality testing. Groups for addicted patients are advantageous because their members share the common homogeneous issue of dealing with addiction as a jump-off point to discussing other problems that may also be shared.

A variety of group formats have been found useful including assertiveness training groups, couples groups, and groups for self-control, ego strength, self-concept, and mood problems (e.g., anxiety, depression). Groups may be used to aid in problem solving, to focus on specific behavioral problems, and to help the patient see that others have similar issues. Groups may be psychodynamically oriented, problem-solving oriented, or confrontation oriented; they may offer couples therapy or occupational counseling. Treatment programs frequently employ orientation didactic groups, which may aid retention in treatment, promote cohesiveness, and support acceptance of longer-term rehabilitation. Although groups are commonly used for alcohol users, they may be especially effective for relapse prevention in cocaine dependence.

Network Therapy

The network therapy approach develops a support group that is tailored to the patient involving family and friends who are not addicted themselves. Network therapy uses a CBT approach regarding triggers; it uses community reinforcement, and support of the patient's social network is essential (19). It can be a useful adjunct to individual therapy or AA and involves psychoeducation of the patient's circle of support about addictions.

Family Evaluation and Therapy

A family evaluation is warranted for all SUD patients; information and aid from the family is crucial for both diagnosis and therapy. Family members are frequently greatly affected by the patient's problems. The family system is often made to accommodate the patient's drinking and may to some degree reinforce it. Confrontation by family members in many cases prompts the patient to seek treatment and may be important in helping the patient continue with treatment.

Family treatment is frequently indicated, especially in families in which considerable support is available to the patient. Children of alcoholics may benefit from family evaluation and treatment.

Family treatments based on the concept of the alcoholic system focus on the correction of dysfunctional patterns of interactional behavior within the family and measure success not only by the achievement of abstinence for the patient but also by the improvement in the level of functioning in the family. Techniques used by family therapists include conjoint family therapy, marital therapy groups, and conjoint hospitalization for marital couples; the efficacy of these techniques has been documented (20).

Self-Help

Every clinician needs to be thoroughly familiar with the work of the 12-step self-help programs: AA, Al-Anon, NA, Substance Anonymous, Cocaine Anonymous, Gamblers Anonymous, and Overeaters Anonymous (including the personal experience of having attended meetings of both AA and Al-Anon to be in touch with their patients' experiences). There is a small but growing body of evidence documenting the efficacy of AA. Self-help may also be very important for treating cocaine abuse and dependence. Peer-led groups are also helpful (21).

AA was formed in 1935 by Bill Wilson and Dr. Robert Smith in Akron, Ohio, in part as a result of lack of available medical treatment for alcoholism. It had roots in the Oxford movement (later the moral rearmament movement) and a Jungian emphasis on spirituality, and it has grown into an international network that includes more than 2 million members in the United States and 185,000 groups worldwide. The major message of the organization is that people with alcohol use disorders, through recognition of alcoholism as an illness, can achieve sobriety together through a spiritual program that includes accepting powerlessness over alcohol and dependency on some intervention beyond the self. It is a voluntary self-supporting fellowship that avoids any self-serving political or economic activity. Al-Anon is a program parallel to AA that includes self-help for the family. Other family-oriented programs include Alateen, which is a program for teenage users and teenage children of alcoholics, and groups for adult children of alcoholics.

How It Works

A 12-step program involves a series of steps and traditions that rely heavily on self-honesty, sobriety, group process, humility, provision of successful role models, self-care, and destigmatization of alcoholism as an illness. Although a 12-step program is frequently recommended in conjunction with a variety of other treatment approaches, for many patients the program may suffice as the sole treatment for an SUD. On average, members attend approximately four meetings per week, although in the early stages of involvement, many attend 90 meetings in 90 days. Patients with multiple addictions may attend several different 12-step programs. A variety of types of meetings include open ones that the interested public may attend, closed meetings, meetings for new members, discussion groups, and homogeneous groups. Although groups vary in style, most generally have a warm, family feel and provide a sense of acceptance, mutual help, and understanding. The assumption is that alcoholics intuitively understand and can identify with universal problems faced by other alcoholics and can share feelings in a group. An emphasis on mutual help through helping others with the same problem has contributed widely to the success of this group, and a large part of the spirituality of the program is embedded in the generosity in time and energy of its members. A system of sponsorship of members by veteran AA members and the creation of a support network of exchanged telephone numbers are important aspects of AA membership. AA provides an opportunity for people to practice relatedness, gain structure, test values, test judgment, practice honesty, find acceptance, and regain hope.

New Developments in 12-Step Programs

Although AA began solely for patients with alcoholism and originally comprised mostly white middle-class men, many more members of AA are women. Also, many alcoholics seek help earlier in their illness. An expansion into a younger population having more dual addictions and additional psychiatric problems has led to greater attention to groups and their specific needs. Subgroups have developed for alcoholics who are gay and lesbian, physicians, adult children of alcoholics, atheists and agnostics, HIV positive, and those with dual diagnosis. Meetings can be found in major cities throughout the world and are essential for alcoholics who travel.

Referrals to 12-Step Programs

The therapist may take an active role in referring a patient to 12-step programs in addition to monitoring and interpreting resistances to regular attendance. The physician can have the patient call AA directly from the office or may call for the patient in order to select a meeting. A phone number (or Web site) for AA intergroup is easily obtainable, and volunteers are glad to provide information about AA. Clinicians should address concerns of or negative responses felt by patients during their first AA meetings. Initially, patients may have difficulties understanding AA or may be socially avoidant. Patients with reactions to the spirituality of AA, who feel criticized in AA because they take psychiatric medications, or who do not feel accepted because of a history of polysubstance abuse will need explanation and support. Patients should be encouraged to get an AA sponsor.

Counseling

Certified alcohol and drug counselors have increasingly played prominent roles in alcohol and drug treatment programs. Counselors are involved in every phase of treatment, including evaluation, psychoeducation, individual and group counseling, and aftercare. For relapse prevention, counselors frequently provide support, advice, and valuable information regarding treatment and 12-step programs.

Education

Most programs include education about the effects of alcohol and drugs, effects on the family, treatment alternatives, and relapse prevention. Education reduces fear, guilt, and shame, supports the medical model, and provides hope. Lectures, discussion groups, films, books, and homework assignments are an important part of the work of treatment and help keep patients productively engaged during treatment.

Psychopharmacological Modalities

In the treatment of SUDs, medications may be prescribed for detoxification, treatment of comorbid psychiatric disorders, complicated neuropsychological and medical disorders, aversive treatment (e.g., disulfiram in alcoholics), attenuation of craving or euphoria (e.g., naltrexone), or psychological ego support. Generally, these medications are used as adjuncts to psychosocial treatment and education. Physicians should have a clear understanding of differential diagnosis and history of substance abuse disorders, the limitations of medications, drug-drug interactions, and side effects.

Naltrexone

For alcohol relapse prevention, the superior efficacy of naltrexone (Revia) for alcohol relapse prevention is well documented (22). It usually prevents relapse when it is given at 50 mg/day for 3 months. Opioid-receptor functioning is thought to be related to the etiology of alcohol dependence. Opioid mu-receptor antagonists decrease overall alcohol use, most likely by blocking release of dopamine in the nucleus accumbens.

Naltrexone's original indication was in the prevention of opioid relapse. As an opioid receptor antagonist, it causes withdrawal symptoms in patients experiencing opioid intoxication, and thus protocols have been used to slowly administer this medication in conjunction with outpatient clonidine treatment for withdrawal. These protocols are summarized in Table 8–7. The main indication of naltrexone is for daily relapse prevention, usually at 50 mg/day.

Methadone and LAAM

Methadone has a dose-dependent effect on concurrent use of opioids and cocaine, and high doses (65 mg/day) may be most effective. A stable dose need not be altered except in the case of changes in pharmacokinetics due to emesis; use of phenytoin, rifampin, barbiturates, carbamazepine, and tricyclic antidepressants; heavy labor; or alcohol intoxication. LAAM is a long-acting opioid agonist with similar uses to methadone for maintenance. It has a longer half-life and thus may be taken only 3 times a week.

Buprenorphine

Buprenorphine (Buprenex) is a mixed opioid agonist-antagonist that is more effective than placebo in the treatment of opioid dependence (23). Buprenorphine shows promise for both opiate detoxification and maintenance. A buprenorphine/naloxone 4:1 combination sublingual tablet is close to FDA approval for use in opiate detoxification and maintenance. The naloxone in the tablet discourages illegal injection street use because it precipitates withdrawal. The regulation of the use of buprenorphrine will, it is hoped, allow greater access of treatment compared to methadone because individual physicians will qualify to prescribe it.

Disulfiram

Disulfiram (Antabuse) is a medication adjunct in the treatment of recovering alcoholics. It is used as aversive treatment to enhance motivation for continued abstinence by making the alcohol-induced high unavailable, thus discouraging impulsive alcohol use. Disulfiram is a potent reversible aldehyde dehydrogenase inhibitor. Aldehyde dehydrogenase is an enzyme that metabolizes acetaldehyde, the first metabolite of alcohol. Inhibition of this metabolic step produces a buildup of acetaldehyde, resulting in toxicity, which consists of nausea, vomiting, cramps, flushing, and vasomotor collapse. Disulfiram has relatively mild side effects, including sedation, halitosis, skin rash, and temporary impotence. More serious side effects, which include peripheral neuropathy, seizures, optic neuritis, and psychosis, occur rarely. Disulfiram also appears to have a catecholamine effect, which may contribute to its reaction with alcohol and make its use contraindicated with monoamine oxidase inhibitor (MAOI) use. It also may inhibit the metabolism of other medications including anticoagulants, phenytoin, and isoniazid, which leads to higher than expected serum levels of these medications. The drug also has adverse interactions with cough syrups. It should be avoided in patients with hepatic disease peripheral neuropathy, renal failure, and cardiac disease and in patients who are pregnant. Other contraindications include medical conditions that would be greatly exacerbated by a disulfiram-alcohol reaction, including liver disease, esophageal varices, heart disease, heart failure, emphysema, and peptic ulcer disease. It should be avoided in anyone likely to become pregnant. Psychiatric contraindications include psychosis and severe depression. Disulfiram can exacerbate psychosis; depressed suicidal patients may purposely precipitate a disulfiram reaction.

Initial doses of disulfiram are 250–500 mg/day. It can be administered in an oral suspension. Subcutaneous implantation is not clinically available. Dosages can be decreased to 125 mg if sedation or other side effects are excessive or in cases with relative contraindications. Patients should be informed about the rationale of disulfiram use, the disulfiram-alcohol reaction, and common side effects.

Treatment facilities vary in their use and attitudes toward disulfiram. Some AA-oriented programs may discourage the use of any medication and consider disulfiram to be an unnecessary psychopharmacological crutch. Many programs use disulfiram as an adjunctive tool in promoting abstinence. Although there has not been convincing evidence that disulfiram use affects long-term outcomes globally, disulfiram has been shown to be useful in certain subtypes of alcoholism, often when it can be administered by a significant other. The best candidates for disulfiram use are adult, socially stable alcoholics and affluent, married, less sociopathic patients who tend to be compulsive.

Lithium

Lithium is an integral component in the treatment of SUDs that have underlying primary bipolar or cyclothymic disorders. Lithium may mute or abort extreme mood swings or indirectly affect substance intake. Mania or hypomania is associated with increased alcohol or cocaine use. Lithium-responsive depression may also be associated with cocaine or alcohol abuse. Lithium has also been associated with decreased subjective experience of intoxication, antagonization of deficits in cognitive and motor function during intoxication, and reduced alcohol consumption. Caution should be exercised in prescribing lithium to patients who are actively abusing substances or who demonstrate poor compliance with treatment; these patients should be hospitalized to ensure abstinence and titration of a proper dose. There are no known uses of lithium in uncomplicated alcohol abuse or dependence. For adolescents with bipolar disorder and secondary substance dependence disorder, lithium is an efficacious treatment for both (24).

Valproic Acid

Valproic acid is used in the treatment of bipolar disorder. Moderate doses of valproate (with an average blood level of approximately 70 mg/L) in alcoholics without significant hepatic disease do not cause significant adverse effects on white blood cell count, platelet count, or liver transaminase level (25).

Antidepressants

Antidepressants do not directly alter SUDs but are important adjuncts in the treatment of patients with primary mood disorders. Determining the antidepressant of choice follows considerations of the depressive subtype and side-effect profile of the medications, and the recognition that judgment, impulse control, and cognition may be impaired in alcoholics in early recovery. Extreme caution should be used in placing alcoholics on MAOIs for depression, especially because wine contains tyramine. Also, intoxication may further impair judgment and increase the risk of using tyramine-containing products. There is evidence that fluoxetine is not helpful for primary cocaine dependence. Venlafaxine, a broad spectrum antidepressant, may be a safe, well-tolerated, rapidly acting, and effective treatment for patients with a dual diagnosis of depression and cocaine dependence. Venlafaxine's potential to cause diastolic hypertension at higher doses indicates monitoring of blood pressure.

Dopamimetics

Bromocriptine has been studied in the treatment of cocaine addiction. It had been hypothesized that because the effects of cocaine are dopamine related and because dopamine depletion was associated with cocaine craving, a dopamimetic substance such as bromocriptine may have some value in the acute onset of abstinence (first 3–4 days) by diminishing cocaine craving. However, studies have failed to justify application of bromocriptine, and psychiatrists do not recommend its use in cocaine SUDs. Similarly, amantadine has not been found to aid in cocaine dependence.

Clonidine

The use of clonidine in opioid detoxification is discussed above. Clonidine has also been reported to be helpful in alcohol withdrawal. There have been case reports of the successful use of clonidine for patients with hallucinogen persisting perception disorder (26).

Carbamazepine

Although previously felt to be helpful for symptoms that result from cocaine abstinence, recent studies have failed to find carbamazepine to be an effective agent against cocaine (27).

Adrenergic Blockades

Using propranolol, a beta-blocker, to reduce adrenergic signs in alcohol withdrawal is controversial and not routinely advocated. Beta-blockers are contraindicated in cocaine intoxication and withdrawal.

Neuroleptics

Neuroleptics have no place in the treatment of primary alcoholism. Use of neuroleptics lowers the seizure threshold and has the long-term risk of tardive dyskinesia. However, neuroleptics can be very helpful in treating patients with psychosis for a wide spectrum of toxic drug reactions. They can be used adjunctively with benzodiazepines in the treatment of delirium, including d.t.'s. Neuroleptics are the primary treatment of choice for patients with alcohol hallucinosis. Among the newer neuroleptics, olanzapine appears to be as effective as haloperidol in the treatment of cannabis-induced psychotic disorder, and it is associated with a lower rate of extrapyramidal symptoms (28).

Benzodiazepines

Benzodiazepines are the drug of choice for treatment of alcohol or benzodiazepine detoxification. They work through the GABA receptor and are very effective in suppressing anxiety symptoms. They also produce tolerance with psychological and physical dependence. Benzodiazepines are generally contraindicated in any SUD except when used for detoxification, acutely for manic patients, or very selectively in compliant abstinent patients with anxiety disorders when other treatments have failed.

The SUD patient who has an underlying anxiety disorder, often with high-dose benzodiazepine abuse, presents a common dilemma. These patients may have a relapse of symptoms on detoxification from CNS depressants. It is often difficult to distinguish among underlying disorders, anxiety symptoms associated with chronic subacute withdrawal, reactive fear, and anxiety about withdrawal. After detoxification, SUD patients with anxiety disorders may be extremely anxious and dysphoric; temptations to relieve this suffering may lead clinicians to reinstate addictive substances, which can lead to a poor outcome. Effective utilization of other, perhaps more specific, treatment modalities including selective serotonin reuptake inhibitors (SSRIs), desipramine, or MAOIs for panic disorder; neuroleptics for psychotic disorders; and SSRIs, buspirone, gabapentin, and adrenergic blockers for generalized anxiety. Setting firm limits on the use of psychoactive substances is necessary. Nonetheless, sometimes benzodiazepines can be a treatment of last resort in compliant anxious patients who maintain sobriety.

Buspirone

Buspirone (BuSpar) is a new anxiolytic with no CNS depressant activity. Clinical studies have so far demonstrated little abuse potential or withdrawal syndrome. It apparently does not potentiate the effects of alcohol. Buspirone is a useful adjunct in the treatment of generalized anxiety or transient anxiety in some substance abusers. Buspirone has the disadvantage of slow onset of efficacy (up to 3 weeks); it is thus of little use in transient anxiety disorders.

Acamprosate

Acamprosate is a very promising drug in alcohol relapse prevention (29). It crosses the blood-brain barrier, is chemically similar to amino acid neurotransmitters, and acts at the *N*-methyl-D-aspartate receptor to reduce the glutaminergic hyperactivity of withdrawal. It is dose dependent and has no abuse potential. Giving acamprosate to those dependent on alcohol will not lead to an acute withdrawal syndrome. Acamprosate is not metabolized but is renally excreted and should be given with caution to those with renal disease. A starting dose is 2–3 g/day in divided doses. Common side effects include diarrhea or headache.

Ondansetron

Ondansetron, a selective serotonin-3 receptor antagonist, has shown promise in reducing alcohol intake in general, specifically among Type I alcoholics, and in diminishing the subjective positive effects of alcohol. Its widespread use is dependent on results of further study.

■ SPECIAL ISSUES IN TREATMENT

Treatment of Mentally Ill, Chemically Abusing Patients

Most psychiatric patients have more than one psychiatric diagnosis, and the most frequent comorbid diagnoses are SUDs. Every patient with an SUD needs a careful psychiatric assessment and treatment plan. Conversely, a thorough substance use history is an essential part of all psychiatric interviews. Interactions between SUDs and other psychiatric diagnoses must be integrated into treatment planning. SUDs are comorbid with disorders of mood, anxiety, personality, and sexual orientation and with organic disorders, schizophrenia, and anorexia nervosa. SUDs can mask, mimic, or result from a wide variety of psychiatric and medical disorders. The psychiatrist provides an understanding of SUDs in relation to other psychiatric illness and determines the course of action at the most appropriate level, be it psychosocial or medical.

Longitudinal, adoption, epidemiological, and family studies have not yet settled old questions as to the cause, effect, or coexistent relationship between psychopathology and addictive behavior. Most studies support the idea that the inherited predisposition to addiction is independent of other psychiatric disorders. The trait of addiction may be primary to psychiatric illness, develop as a way of coping with other problems, or coexist with other psychiatric disorders. Treatment planning for patients with psychiatric disorders depends on flexibility and a broad understanding of psychiatry and of alcohol and drug abuse.

The Challenging Patient With Dual Diagnosis

Complex interactions between psychopathology and addiction are hard to separate clinically because of overlapping signs and symptoms that result from intoxication, withdrawal, mixed drug reactions, adverse drug responses, medical conditions, and the organic and psychosocial effects of substance use on affective state, anxiety, or personality. The addition of other Axis I, II, and III disorders complicates diagnoses and makes treatment more difficult. Also, treating addictions in patients with psychiatric illness is complicated by risk of violence toward self or others associated with anxiety; irritation, anger, impulsivity, and poor reality testing in patients experiencing intoxication or withdrawal; and aggressivity resulting from use of cocaine, hallucinogens, PCP, or alcohol.

Personnel in the mental health field and the substance abuse field should have the rudimentary knowledge to screen patients properly and to develop a treatment plan that adequately addresses the patient's needs. Model programs have been developed around the country to integrate psychiatric and substance abuse treatments. However, the dual-diagnosis patient often falls through the cracks of the treatment system. Severe psychiatric disorders often preclude full treatment in substance abuse clinics or self-help groups. Confrontational techniques and self-exposure, as done in some substance abuse programs, may exacerbate psychiatric symptoms. Special AA and NA groups are being formed for dual-diagnosis or so-called double trouble patients. Patients with severe psychiatric illness benefit significantly from additional professional psychiatric therapy. Some patients, especially patients with frank psychosis or suicidal ideation, require primary psychiatric settings (e.g., day hospital or inpatient setting). However, treatment for primary psychiatric disorders should not preclude addressing substance abuse issues. Attendance at AA or NA meetings should be arranged if possible. An addiction psychiatrist should be available to psychiatric facilities with a high number of dual-diagnosis patients. The addiction psychiatrist may be best included as part of a multidisciplinary team approach.

A discussion of treatment of dual-diagnosis patients would not be complete without the recognition of some of the pressing social needs of these patients. Often these patients have alienated family, friends, and treatment personnel. The need for adequate housing, health, and follow-up is imperative. Residential facilities are needed to ease the transition of dual-diagnosis patients into society. Coordination of the various agencies is needed. Talbott discussed the case management approach extensively (30). There is evidence that wrap-around care, or integrated care, helps (31). Often, however, substance abuse facilities refuse admission to psychiatric patients, and psychiatric facilities refuse patients with a history of substance abuse.

Careful consideration must be given to psychiatric patients who abuse drugs when it comes to choosing psychopharmacological treatment with medications that are themselves abusable. For example, patients with attention-deficit/hyperactivity disorder who abuse cocaine are at high risk for treatment failure or dropout. Notwithstanding plausible controversy over the use of stimulants in substance abusers, use of sustained-release methylphenidate (Ritalin) may help these patients.

Rehabilitation

The rehabilitation model, pioneered in treatment of SUDs, has become an important model for a variety of categories of psychiatric illness. It combines self-help, counseling, education, relapse prevention, group treatment, a warm supportive environment, and emphasis on a medical model geared to reducing stigma and blame. Most treatment units are highly structured, insist on an abstinence goal, and use lectures, films, and discussion groups as part of a complete cognitive and educational program. Patients are frequently converted into active 12-step members and are encouraged to continue in aftercare.

A highly skilled professional team with available consultation is needed to integrate counseling; cognitive and behavioral treatment; relapse prevention strategies; interpersonal, family, and group therapy; applied or brief psychodynamically oriented psychotherapy; social network approaches; education; and occupational and recreational therapy. Inpatient programs previously included 5–7 days for detoxification and 3–6 weeks for rehabilitation, but now parts of the programs are often sited in halfway houses in outpatient settings, and hospital stays of 3–12 days are more common. Longer stays are indicated for adolescents, as well as for patients with greater severity of illness, dual diagnoses, or severe medical problems.

The rehabilitation model emphasizes providing opportunities for patients to practice social skills, gain control over impulses, and use the highly structured program as an auxiliary superego, and it encourages self-honesty and expression of feelings. The program promotes the use of higher-level defenses (e.g., intellectualization) and actively confronts more primitive defenses (e.g., denial, splitting, and projection), especially when these defenses are used in relation to the issue of abstinence (32).

Rehabilitation can take place in freestanding rehabilitation programs, mental illness–chemical abuse units, general hospitals, inpatient programs, organized outpatient day and evening hospitals, therapeutic communities, and halfway houses. Addiction day treatment programs utilize many of the same techniques employed in inpatient treatment programs. Addiction day treatment programs are staffed by interdisciplinary teams that develop individualized treatment plans. Organized outpatient alcohol programs may provide a range of treatment modalities with varying intensity. Outpatient programs are less restrictive, provide an alternative to hospitalization, and may be useful as part of an aftercare program.

Aftercare

Patient aftercare is necessary on discharge from an inpatient or organized outpatient program. Referral to a 12-step program often complements other treatment, although self-help may suffice for some faithfully attending people. At least 2 years of follow-up after start of abstinence is recommended.

■ REFERENCES

1. Armour D, Polich J, Stambul H: Alcoholism and Treatment. New York, Wiley, 1978
2. Marlatt G, Gordon J: Relapse Prevention. New York, Guilford Press, 1985
3. Perry S, Frances A, Clarkin J: A DSM-III-R Casebook of Treatment Selection. New York, Brunner/Mazel, 1984

4. McLellan AT, Grissom GR, Zanis D, et al: Problem-service matching in addiction treatment: a prospective study in 4 programs. Arch Gen Psychiatry 54:730–735, 1997

5. Acute reactions to drugs of abuse. Medical Letter 38:43–46, 1996

6. Goldberg MJ, Spector R, Park GD, et al: An approach to the management of the poisoned patient. Arch Intern Med 146:1381–1385, 1986

7. Sullivan JT, Sykora K, Schneiderman J, et al: Assessment of alcohol withdrawal: the revised Clinical Institute Withdrawal Assessment for Alcohol Scale (CIWA-Ar). B J Addict 84:1353–1377, 1989

8. O'Connor PG, Waugh ME, Carrol KM, et al: Primary care-based ambulatory opioid detoxification: the results of a clinical trial. J Gen Intern Med 10:255–260, 1995

9. O'Connor PG, Carroll KM, Shi JM, et al: Three methods of opioid detoxification in a primary care setting: a randomized trial. Ann Intern Med 127:526–530, 1997

10. Ling W, Charuvastra C, Collins JF, et al: Buprenorphine maintenance treatment of opiate dependence: a multicenter, randomized clinical trial. Addiction 93:475–486, 1998

11. Hernandez-Avila CA, Ortega-Soto HA, Jasso A, et al: Treatment of inhalant-induced psychotic disorder with carbamazepine versus haloperidol. Psychiatr Serv 49:812–815, 1998

12. American Psychiatric Association: Practice guideline for the treatment of patients with nicotine dependence. Am J Psychiatry 153 (suppl 10):1–31, 1996

13. Anton RF, Moak DH, Waid LR, et al: Naltrexone and cognitive behavioral therapy for the treatment of outpatient alcoholics: results of a placebo-controlled trial. Am J Psychiatry 156:1758–1764, 1999

14. Frances R, Borg L, Mack A, et al: Individual treatment: psychodynamics and the treatment of substance-related disorders, in Treatments of Psychiatric Disorders, 3rd Edition. Edited by Gabbard G. Washington, DC, American Psychiatric Publishing, 2001

15. Wright FD, Beck AT, Newman CF, et al: Cognitive therapy of substance abuse: theoretical rationale. NIDA Res Monogr 137:123–146, 1993

16. Linehan MM, Schmidt H III, Dimeff LA, et al: Dialectical behavior therapy for patients with borderline personality disorder and drug-dependence. Am J Addict 8:279–292, 1999

17. Samet JH, Rollnick S, Barnes H: Beyond CAGE: a brief clinical approach after detection of substance abuse. Arch Intern Med 156:2287–2293, 1990

18. Prochaska JO, DiClemente CC, Norcross JC: In search of how people change: applications to addictive behavior. Am Psychol 47:1102–1114, 1992

19. Galanter M, Keller D, Dermatis H: Network therapy for addiction: assessment of the clinical outcome of training. Am J Psychiatry 150:28–36, 1993

20. Edwards ME, Steinglass P: Family therapy treatment outcomes for alcoholism. J Marital Fam Ther 21:475–509, 1995

21. Galanter M: Self help treatment for combined addiction and mental illness. Hospital and Community Psychiatry 51:877–879, 2000

22. Volpicelli JR, Alterman AI, Hayashida M, et al: Naltrexone in the treatment of alcohol dependence. Arch Gen Psychiatry 49:876–887, 1992

23. Johnson RE, Eissenberg T, Stitzer ML, et al: A placebo controlled clinical trial of buprenorphine as a treatment for opioid dependence. Drug Alcohol Depend 40:17–25, 1995

24. Geller B, Cooper TB, Sun K, et al: Double-blind and placebo-controlled study of lithium for adolescent bipolar disorders with secondary substance dependency. J Am Acad Child Adolesc Psychiatry 37:171–178, 1998

25. Sonne S, Brady KY: Valproate for alcoholics with bipolar disorder. Am J Psychiatry 156:1122, 1999

26. Lerner AG, Finkel B, Oyfee I, et al: Clonidine treatment for hallucinogen persisting perception disorder. Am J Psychiatry 155:1460, 1998

27. Cornish JW, Maany I, Fudala PJ, et al: Carbamazepine treat-

ment for cocaine dependence. Drug Alcohol Depend 38:221–227, 1995

28. Berk M, Brook S, Trandafir AI: A comparison of olanzapine with haloperidol in cannabis-induced psychotic disorder: a double-blind randomized controlled trial. Int Clin Psychopharmacol 14:177–180, 1999

29. Sass H, Soyka M, Mamm K, et al: Relapse prevention by acamprosate: results from a placebo-controlled study on alcohol dependence. Arch Gen Psychiatry 53:673–680, 1996

30. Talbott J (ed): The Chronic Mentally Ill: Treatment, Programs, Systems. New York, Human Sciences Press, 1981

31. Ries RK, Comtois KA: Illness severity and treatment services for dually diagnosed severely mentally ill outpatients. Schizophr Bull 23:239–246, 1997

32. Frances RJ, Alexopoulos GS: The inpatient treatment of the alcoholic patient. Psychiatric Annals 12:386–391, 1982

9

TREATMENT APPROACHES IN SPECIFIC POPULATIONS

■ WOMEN

In the United States, the ratio of alcoholism in men compared with women is 3:1. However, the ratio is generally 1:1 for other substance use disorders (SUDs) (except for prescription drugs, which are disproportionately used by women) (1). Women are underrepresented in treatment programs, and their special needs are often not addressed during treatment. However, the stigma of SUDs affects women gravely; women suffer greater medical morbidity secondary to addictions than men (2). Traditionally, women with SUDs are identified differently from men. Violence or other reckless behavior often brings men with SUDs to the attention of family, friends, and treatment personnel. Women abusers are mostly discovered through nonviolent situations, such as their employee assistance programs (EAPs), through family interventions, or in obstetric/gynecological evaluations. (However, recent data show that more women who abuse substances are violent than was previously thought [3]). The possibilities of fetal alcohol syndrome and HIV transmission contribute greater urgency to identification of alcoholism and intravenous drug use in women. Women more frequently present with coexisting panic, anxiety, mood, and eating disorders than do men, and women less frequently have accompanying antisocial problems. Women who experience sexual abuse in childhood often develop alcohol and drug abuse problems as adults. Women suffer greatly from and are profoundly affected by the abuse of fathers and husbands with alcoholism. Women who abuse alcohol have a later age at onset of substance abuse and a more rapid progression of abuse and consume a smaller amount of alcohol than men who abuse alcohol. They are also more likely than men to have a significant other who is also a substance abuser, and women who abuse alcohol have higher rates of comorbid psychiatric disorders.

Women with alcohol SUDs are also more likely than men to attempt suicide but less likely to complete it. They also tend to have a history of sexual or physical abuse and date the onset of the SUD to a stressful event. Women with alcohol SUDs have a higher mortality rate and are more likely to report previous psychiatric treatment than are men. Women with cocaine SUDs have a more rapid progression of the disease, use less often than men with cocaine SUDs, usually have a spouse who also has an SUD, and have a greater likelihood of suicide attempts than men. Women with cocaine SUDs often have a history of sexual or physical abuse and date the SUD onset to a stressful event.

Genetic, Cultural, and Biological Effects

Most research on the heredity of alcoholism has been done on men. Recent studies indicate that a genetic potential for alcoholism also exists in women, although it may very well be that this is frequently overridden by cultural influences. Alcoholism in women varies markedly depending on the culture. For Koreans, the male to female ratio for alcoholism is 28:1. Women have a higher blood alcohol level (BAL) pound per pound per drink compared with men, and their BAL is affected differently at different times in the menstrual cycle. Women are most frequently admitted to alcohol treatment hospitals during the perimenstrual time, which is often marked by heavier drinking. In addition to a lower tolerance for alcohol, women tend to have a more telescoped course of the chronic effects of excessive drinking, including cirrhosis of the liver, compared with men. The differences between alcoholism in men and women may be partially explained by the fact that men have greater amounts of alcohol dehydrogenase in the gastric mucosa. Alcohol and drugs in women may initially be used to reduce sexual inhibitions; however, ultimately alcohol reduces desire and ability to perform sexually in women, as in men, and recovery usually leads to better sexual function.

Psychiatric Comorbidity

Women with SUDs have mood disorders more commonly than men. In fact, with the exception of attention-deficit disorder and antisocial personality disorder, women experience increased comorbid psychopathology, particularly for anxiety disorders (especially posttraumatic stress disorder) and eating disorders (4). Secondary alcoholism with self-medication for anxiety or depression is much more frequent in women than in men. Sometimes alcoholism may develop after benzodiazepine dependence, which may have started during efforts to treat anxiety disorders.

Treatment Issues

Women in traditional treatment programs often experience discomfort when talking about sexual abuse and sexual issues in mixed male-female groups. Women may feel intimidated and outnumbered by men in alcohol rehabilitation programs. Thus, women's groups and special programs and residences for women in rehabilitation programs are beneficial. In general, although treatment for alcoholism and drug abuse in women is similar in many ways to treatment for men, tailoring of the treatment is needed to address differences. Special treatment includes an especially close watch for the possibility of sedative-hypnotic dependence, anxiety disorders and depression, extrasensitivity to stigma, and abusive spouses. An awareness of fetal alcohol and drug effects is also stressed. Contact with recovered alcoholic women as role models and work with female professionals may also be a factor in improved self-esteem.

The care of women of childbearing age with SUDs requires a great deal of attention. Careful use of medication in women of childbearing age includes awareness of relative risks and benefits.

Treatment of depression and anxiety disorders in women with dual diagnosis is often necessary. Inpatient treatment poses special problems for young mothers, and few programs exist in which women can be hospitalized along with their children. Alcoholic women have increased fears of loss of custody and increased needs for child-care services. Women frequently have economic problems that may make it more difficult for them to get good treatment. Although alcoholic men are frequently married to nonalcoholic women who are supportive of their husbands' recovery, more often women with alcoholism are married to addicted men who may be less helpful or even negative toward recovery. Women may need to separate from an addicted, abusing spouse to get well and often need help for sobriety from sober women friends and female role models who are in the process of recovery. General aspects of the care of addicted women are given in Table 9–1 (5).

TABLE 9–1. **Special considerations in women's treatment**

Psychiatric assessment for comorbid disorders; date of onset for each (primary/secondary)
Attention to past history and present risk of physical and sexual assault
Assessment of prescription drug abuse/dependence
Comprehensive physical examination for physical complications and comorbid disorders
Need for access to health care (including obstetric care)
Psychoeducation to include information on substance use in pregnancy
Child-care services for women in treatment
Parenting education and assistance
Evaluation and treatment of significant others and children
Positive female role models (among treatment staff, friends, self-help)
Attention to guilt, shame, and self-esteem issues
Assessment and treatment of sexual dysfunction
Attention to the effects of sexism in the previous experience of the patient (for example, underemployment, lack of opportunity, and rigid sex roles)
Avoidance of iatrogenic drug dependence
Special attention to the needs of minority women, lesbian women, and women in the criminal justice system

Problems Secondary to Addiction in Women

General Medical Conditions

Women who abuse substances are at risk of developing a number of specific general medical conditions, and, compared to men, when they develop such secondary conditions, they occur at a faster rate and with higher morbidity, which is called *telescoping*. Alcoholic cardiomyopathy and cirrhosis occur at a faster rate in women than in men (6). Recent studies have found that women who abuse alcohol are at greater risk of developing breast cancer than are women who do not use alcohol (7). Female SUD patients require comprehensive follow-up in the primary care setting.

Acquired Immunodeficiency Syndrome

HIV infection is a growing pandemic whose effects are seen every day among women with SUDs, especially minority women. A majority of women in methadone treatment programs in urban centers are HIV positive; a majority of these women are also mothers. Female prostitution can be another cause of the spread of AIDS and is also frequently associated with intravenous drug use.

A special concern of women is the possibility of contracting AIDS through intercourse with HIV-positive men. Women who use substances may frequently take more risks, have poorer self-care, and less frequently insist on safe sex. Women of childbearing age who are intravenous drug users are at special high risk and need careful counseling.

Effects on Sexual and Reproductive Function

Sexual function is affected by almost all drugs of abuse. Despite its reputation, alcohol is not an aphrodisiac, and all sexually active female alcoholics should be reminded that sexual function improves with sobriety (8). Libido is decreased as a result of cocaine and amphetamine use. Also, heroin disrupts ovulation. The treatment of neonates for methadone withdrawal is a common procedure, and methadone use is not an absolute contraindication to pregnancy (9). Cocaine can cause abruptio placentae and ventricular tachycardia in the neonate (10).

Fetal Alcohol Syndrome

Fetal alcohol syndrome occurs in approximately 1–3 infants per 1,000 live births generally, and as high as 1 in 100 births in some Inuit villages (11). Typical signs of fetal alcohol syndrome include low birth weight, growth deficiency with delayed motor development, mental retardation and learning problems, and other less severe fetal alcohol behavioral effects. No safe alcohol level during pregnancy has been established, and dangers increase with dose used.

■ CHILDREN AND ADOLESCENTS

The use, abuse, prevention, and treatment of SUDs in children and adolescents are of grave concern, and the prevalence of SUDs in this group is rising, the age of first usage is dropping, and the morbidity and mortality of children and adolescents with SUDs are increasing. Substance abuse can interfere with natural growth and normal interaction and development, including relationships with peers, performance in school, attitudes toward law and authority, and acute and chronic organic effects. The question of when use becomes abuse and dependency in adolescents is controversial. There is a continuum between hazardous harmful use and abuse. It is more difficult to diagnose dependence in adolescents because of the reduced likelihood of signs and symptoms of withdrawal that frequently occur later in addiction. Adolescents are less likely to report withdrawal symptoms, have shorter periods of addiction, and may recover more rapidly from withdrawal symptoms. Early identification of patterns of drug use that interfere with relationships, school performance, and ability to provide good self-care are important in addition to physiological symptoms of tolerance and withdrawal. There are specific practice parameters for the treatment of SUDs in children and adolescents (12).

Extent of the Problem

According to the latest figures from the Substance Abuse and Mental Health Services Administration (SAMHSA) national household survey, drug abuse by adolescents (12–17 years old) decreased slightly between 1997 and 1999 from 11.4% to 9.9% to 9.0%. However, this follows a stark increase in abuse that occurred starting in 1992, when the rate of past month use among youth ages 12–17 had reached a low of 5.3% from a high of 16.3% in 1979. Since 1995, when the rate had climbed to 10.9%, the rate has fluctuated from 9% to 11% (see www.samhsa.gov/OAS/NHSDA/98Summ). Furthermore, the age at which drugs or alcohol is used first has dropped such that more than 50% of sixth graders have tried alcohol or other illicit substances (13). Racial and ethnic differences are apparent among this population: African American children use the least, Hispanic children use the most in the eighth grade, and whites use most in twelfth grade. However, Hispanics disproportionately use more cocaine, heroin, and steroids in twelfth grade than do other groups (14). Thus the problem of youth substance use is wide, growing, and complex.

Early Detection in Adolescents

Signs of adolescent drug use include a drop in school performance, irritability, apathy, mood change (including depression), poor self-care, weight loss, oversensitivity with regard to questions about drinking or drugs, and sudden changes in friends. Screening devices for adolescents should include routine medical examinations before camp or in school. The use of urine analysis may help confirm a diagnosis when necessary. Efforts at early detection of substance use are vital because it is increasingly recognized that a younger age at onset of addiction is associated with a poorer outcome, including alcohol-related harm, and early detection has a greater potential for clinically significant use (15).

Contributing Factors

Peer group, school environment, age, geography, race, values, family attitudes toward substance abuse, risk-seeking temperament, and biological predisposition are all contributing factors to adolescent substance abuse. Nonuser adolescents are more likely to describe close relationships with their parents than are users. Adolescents who do not use substances are more likely to be comfortably dependent on their parents and closer to their family than users, who report themselves as independent and distant. Users more frequently indicate that they do not want to be like their parents, do not feel they need their parents' approval, and do not acknowledge a desire for affection from their parents. Frequently, there is a positive family history for chemical dependence in adolescents with substance abuse problems. Genetic studies indicate a strong hereditary predisposition to alcoholism. If children do not abuse substances by age 21, they are unlikely to do so after that point.

Families

In SUD treatment, the role of the family is more important to adolescent substance abusers than it is to adult substance abusers. However, parents and family members of adolescent abusers may be less resistant to involvement in treatment because they may feel responsible for the adolescent's behavior. When parents themselves are actively addicted, the challenges of treatment are greater. Adolescents are less likely to enter treatment to avoid incarceration than are adults and are likely to be pushed into treatment by their families, schools, and pediatricians and family physicians. Children of divorce have a great risk of substance abuse.

Residential Treatment

Inpatient or residential treatment for adolescents is indicated for those who have had a drug problem that has interfered with their ability to function in school, work, and home environments and who have been unable to maintain abstinence through outpatient treatment. A low motivation to change, a disruptive home life, high incidence of acting out, involvement with the juvenile justice system, and additional psychiatric or medical problems all may be reasons for inpatient treatment. Depression, suicidality, hyperactivity, chemical dependence, and drug overdoses are additional indicators for inpatient treatment. Adolescents frequently require longer hospital stays than adults because they may have greater dispositional problems, more resistance to treatment, greater difficulty of controlling acting out in outpatient therapy, and greater severity of family problems. The treatment outcome for adolescents is worse than it is for adults. Predictors of completion include greater severity of alcohol abuse; greater abuse of drugs other than alcohol, nicotine, or cannabis; higher degree of internalizing problems; and lower self-esteem (16).

Substance Intoxication or Psychosis

Intoxication with drugs and alcohol in adolescents or children may lead to disinhibition, violence, and medical complications. Strategies for managing drug and alcohol intoxication include a quiet, supportive environment that can lessen the chance that the adolescent or child will act out in a violent manner and sometimes include addition of benzodiazepines or atypical antipsychotics. Support staff may be needed to approach potentially violent adolescents or children and to have an additional quieting effect. Police should be involved if the adolescent or child is carrying a weapon. Emergency room checks for weapons are very important. Avoidance of use of sedatives with adolescent abusers is important because benzodiazepines lead to increased disinhibition and increase the possibility of violent acting out.

Mentally Ill, Chemical-Abusing Adolescents

Although the risks vary by diagnosis, all childhood psychiatric disorders are associated with SUDs. Most adolescents entering inpatient drug and alcohol treatment programs have additional mental health problems, which include conduct disorder, affective disorder, attention-deficit/hyperactivity disorder, anxiety disorders, eating disorders, and other Axis I conditions, as well as frequent characterological diagnosis of passive-aggressive personality, borderline personality disorder, and narcissistic personality disorder. The treatment of attention-deficit disorder with methylphenidate in adolescents significantly reduces risk of developing substance abuse patterns later in life (17).

Suicidal ideation and behavior are important in adolescents and children with SUDs, and careful history-taking regarding suicide attempts and thoughts is crucial. If there is a positive family history of suicide or depression, psychosis, isolation from families and friends, previous suicide attempts, clear-cut plans of suicide attempts, or violent means of carrying out the plan, the risk of suicide is increased. SUDs are major risk factors for suicide among adolescents. Alcohol-related motor vehicle accidents are the leading cause of death among youth ages 15–24. There have also been a rash of recent reports of respiratory depression, coma, and death after excessive bouts of alcohol and use of designer drugs such as ecstasy.

Increased alcohol and drug abuse in adolescents is frequently associated with risk-taking behavior linked to spread of HIV infection (e.g., intravenous drug use, unsafe sexual practices, and increased sexual activity with multiple partners). SUDs in adolescents may also directly and indirectly affect the immune system. Sexual abuse of children and adolescents in families in which one or more members has an SUD is not uncommon, and if a family member is HIV positive, it may also increase risk of HIV spread to adolescents.

Assessment

Assessment of the adolescent drug user must be comprehensive. It requires a careful history of both patient and family, including the place and time drugs are used, the circumstances under which drugs are used, the amount of drug used, and the events and reactions that have occurred as a result of drug use. Parents should be asked about the adolescent's behavior, personality changes, school performance and absenteeism, changes in friends, and presence of rebelliousness, and about the number of occasions they thought their adolescent was intoxicated. Parental and sibling drug use history is also important. Parents' reactions to the adolescent's drug use, whether the adolescent has been confronted about possible drug use, and, if applicable, the adolescent's previous response to confrontation are important. Gathering histories from schools, pediatricians, clergy, and probation officers is also useful. The clinician should be aware of the possibility of denial by the adolescent or his or her family.

Clinical Management Issues

The treatment of adolescents requires both structure and flexibility. Awareness of the possibility of contraband stashes and the necessity for intermittent urine screening are important in inpatient treatment programs to monitor compliance. Most programs rely heavily on a therapeutic milieu with individualized treatment planning. A warm, supportive environment with organized structure increases motivation and maximizes positive interaction with other members of the group. Adolescent programs rely heavily on peer-support groups, family therapy, school, education on drug abuse, and 12-step programs such as Alcoholics Anonymous (AA) and Alateen, vocational programs, patient-staff meetings, and activity therapy. Programs that are most successful with adolescents encourage openness and spontaneous expression of feelings, allow patients to engage in independent decision making, have experienced counselors and staff who help patients solve their problems, use cognitive and behavioral approaches and relaxation techniques, and frequently employ the support of volunteers. Cognitive-behavioral approaches have been modified for adolescents and are an efficacious treatment modality. Treatment manuals are available to help use cognitive-behavioral therapy in adolescents (18).

Psychopharmacology

When considering pharmacological interventions in children and adolescents, great care and attention are absolutely required. Disulfiram is rarely used in adolescents. Withdrawal from alcohol is rarely a clinically significant syndrome in children and adolescents, but when it occurs, it should be monitored and treated as it is for adults.

Relapses

Relapse prevention for adolescents is often more difficult than for adults, and the goal of total abstinence becomes more difficult to achieve. Rules that reject the patient after one instance of drug use are less likely to be effective in adolescent treatment services because the adolescent may be looking for a means of escaping treatment. With adolescents, a slip needs to be understood as a symptom of the problem; the patient should not be rejected because of a relapse. Relapses may lead to adjustment of treatment plans and may require rehospitalization. Discharge planning should include outpatient treatment for drug abuse and frequent attendance at self-help support groups. Frequently, family or group treatments are added to individual treatment, depending on need. Urine screens to detect drug and alcohol use are frequently part of a comprehensive outpatient plan. Adolescents may also need halfway houses, residential treatment centers, and in some instances long-term inpatient psychiatric care.

Prevention

The prevention of child and adolescent substance abuse may be understood in terms of supply and demand. Although identifying those at risk is an important first step, current methods of prevention in children and adolescents avoid stirring interest and curiosity and instead concentrate more on teaching life skills that provide support for self-esteem, social skills, and assertiveness training (19).

■ THE ELDERLY

The true scope of alcohol and drug abuse problems in the geriatric population is unknown. The incidence of alcoholism is lower in the elderly population than in the population at large. A greater and more frequent problem is overuse of prescription drugs and interaction of alcohol and other medications. Diagnosis is often more difficult in the elderly, and denial of problems is frequent. Age-related changes in the pharmacokinetics of drugs with enhanced sensitivity to drugs and use of multiple drugs contribute to more severe consequences of substance abuse in the elderly. Substance abuse in the elderly may have late onset in reaction to the stresses of advanced age, including retirement, loss of spouse and friends, and problems with health. Chronic heavy alcohol and substance abuse often lead to premature death, which may in part account for reduction of incidence of chronic alcoholism in the elderly. In addition to selective survival, it has also been postulated that cohort differences contribute to different patterns of cultural acceptances of substance use in different generations. This hypothesis would be consistent with future increases in geriatric alcoholism. Elderly alcoholics (especially men) are at a very high risk of suicide.

Special Problems in Diagnosis

Alcoholism is less likely to be detected in retired people because impairments in social and occupational functioning may not be as obvious. Elderly alcoholics frequently have fewer antisocial problems, and it may be difficult to distinguish the consequences of substance use from aging itself. Cognitive problems are frequent in the elderly in general. Even though they are accelerated by alcoholism, they may be wrongly attributed to degenerative brain disease. The hazards of heavy alcohol use on sleep, sexual functioning, and cognitive ability potentiate the changes that ordinarily occur with aging and with the use of multiple medications.

Complications

The pharmacokinetic changes that normally accompany aging include a relatively increased volume of distribution, a greater CNS sensitivity to toxic substances, and metabolic changes including a diminished ability of the liver to carry out primary enzymatic degradation. The common polypharmacy of the elderly contributes to this problem. The effects of alcohol on the liver potentiate the possibility of overdose and with some drugs may lead to a more rapid metabolism, which may affect the clinical effectiveness of medications needed by the elderly. The depressant effects of alcohol may further contribute to major depression and cognitive impairment. Some elderly patients experience a loss of tolerance, which leads to more intense effects of alcohol with relatively small doses. The dementia that results from alcoholism is not reversible but does not progress upon cessation of drinking (21). Thiamine deficiency is a common etiology of dementia in elderly alcoholics, and in those cases it should be repleted in a timely fashion lest it progress to Wernicke's encephalopathy.

Treatment Issues

Greater creativity, flexibility, and sensitivity should be given to the needs of the elderly. Geriatric patients may need to be protected from threatening and acting-out behaviors of younger patients. Elderly patients also require somewhat less confrontation, a greater degree of support, and greater attention to work with family members. The consequences of divorce are likely to also be greater in this group, and spouses are less likely to do well if abandoned because of a drinking problem. Table 9–2 offers general guidelines for treating elderly alcoholics.

Prescription Drug Abuse

Abuse of prescription drugs is a common problem in the elderly (22). Polypharmacy and sensitivity to toxic effects frequently lead

---

TABLE 9–2. **Guidelines for caring for the elderly**

Avoid disulfiram
Use short-acting benzodiazepines
Remember that full abstinence is less likely to be achieved
Consider the patient's life experiences
Replete thiamine

---

elderly patients into difficult situations. Not infrequently, cessation of medications may cause an apparent dementia to resolve. Benzodiazepine abuse among women is common, and sleep medications contribute to the problem. Memory problems may lead to unintentional misuse and overuse of prescription drugs. Inadequate explanation of the way medication should be taken and misunderstanding of dosage instructions are other problems. Ambulatory abusers of these medications may require hospitalization in order to discontinue use. Nursing home patients are sometimes overmedicated to reduce disruptiveness and to decrease the need for nursing staff.

■ CHRONIC PATIENTS, DISABLED PATIENTS, AND HOMELESS PATIENTS

Chronic psychoactive substance–dependent patients comprise those with polysubstance abuse, with a wide range of available substances, vast exposure to treatment, and a wide range of demographic characteristics. A common characteristic of chronic psychoactive substance–dependent patients is maladaptive use of drugs over a long period of time (exceeding at least a year) with recurrent disability in physical, social, academic, or vocational functioning. Chronic psychoactive substance–dependent patients are frequently in need of long-term institutional treatment, and a paucity of resources are available for sophisticated, targeted treatment of the multiple challenges these patients frequently confront. Clear effectiveness of specific treatments and combinations of treatments has not been established, even though effective treatments are very much needed for the serious problems posed by this population. Unfortunately, Veterans Administration hospitals have reduced the availability of inpatient care to veterans, which affects many elderly people with SUDs.

The chronic patient may be severely stigmatized, possibly because his or her condition is seen as self-inflicted. However, unlike other maladaptive behavior—such as cigarette smoking (leading to emphysema) or lack of compliance with a low-salt diet (contributing to congestive heart failure)—the self-inflicted aspect of addiction has led to prejudice with regard to allocation of resources and handling of benefits and disability. Chronic psychoactive substance–dependent patients may need a wide range of services and links with other programs in the community. Programs need to be culturally relevant and meet local realities of communities. Highly trained staff with positive attitudes toward treatment are needed for implementing treatment of patients with multiple problems.

Cognitively Impaired Chronic Patients

The cognitive impairment that is associated with chronic alcohol and drug dependence is likely to affect the ability of patients to handle cognitive treatment programs. In addition, patients with Korsakoff's syndrome, alcohol dementia, and other severe complications due to alcoholism and drug abuse may be in need of chronic nursing home care. Many treatment failures in alcohol-treatment and drug-treatment programs are based on unrecognized difficulties that patients have in processing information.

Patients With Chronic Mental Illness and Substance Abuse

Chronic mental illness frequently contributes to the chronicity and severity of substance abuse problems. Facilities that combine psychiatric treatment with substance abuse rehabilitation treatment are often not available to patients with chronic mental illness. Severely disturbed drug abusers may be shunned by drug rehabilitation facilities not equipped to handle them. Confrontational methods and overemphasis on a drug-free model, which in some facilities includes underprescribing of psychotropic medication, can be detrimental to the mentally ill.

Chronic Substance Abuse in Those With Multiple and Physical Disabilities

Alcohol and drug abuse may contribute to the development of another physical disability, such as paraplegia or head trauma. The physically disabled patient may have easier access to prescription drugs, and physicians may too readily prescribe medication out of a sense of guilt or futility. Disabled individuals who feel frustrated and angry at being dependent, socially isolated, and discriminated against by the rest of society may be more vulnerable to depression, anxiety, and self-hatred and may have low motivation and low self-esteem. They are more likely to suffer from chronic pain, which may lead to iatrogenic addiction.

Blind and Deaf Patients

Blind and visually impaired patients may have problems coping with their impairment, which may contribute to substance abuse. Deaf patients may have greater denial of the existence of substance abuse problems within their community, are afraid of stigmatization in having an additional problem, and have a lack of adequate signs in sign language to symbolize drunkenness or sobriety. Innovative treatment programs using simultaneous translators in groups to mainstream deaf patients through alcohol rehabilitation programs have been developed. Unfortunately, there are few alcohol and drug counselors who are well trained in sign language and not enough translators who can facilitate communication with such patients.

Paraplegic Patients

The problems of alcohol and drug abuse in patients with spinal cord disabilities are significant. Spinal cord disabilities may have been originally caused by alcohol and substance abuse; physical problems such as decubitus ulcers are caused by immobility and poor nutrition, which may be worsened by substance abuse. Programs need to be geared to treat alcoholic patients with spinal cord disabilities with physical rehabilitation, group psychotherapy, and 12-step recovery groups such as AA and Narcotics Anonymous (NA).

The Mentally Disabled Substance Abuser

Mildly mentally disabled patients (IQ 60–85) are predictable, are concrete thinkers, are easily manipulated, and may have problems learning from experience. Most mildly mentally disabled patients live in the community and may attempt to socialize in neighborhood bars viewed as warm and nonjudgmental. Mentally disabled patients may wish to feel accepted as part of a group, and alcohol and substance use are seen as a means of improving socialization. Treatment and prevention efforts need to take into account the special needs of this population. Poor verbal skills may make it more difficult for them to benefit from AA and NA meetings and group programs that involve cognitive approaches and education about drug abuse. An emphasis on provision of a high degree of acceptance, warmth, and emotional support in working with mentally disabled patients is necessary. If the patients are able to learn that they cannot drink safely and if simple messages of not drinking are reinforced, then they may do very well in treatment.

Homeless Patients With Addictions

Evidence shows that the homeless population is no longer principally composed of "skid row" alcoholics or single, older, chronic alcoholic men (23). The population has been getting younger and includes an increasing number of women; as many as 90% have a primary psychiatric diagnosis. In several different urban samples in the United States, 20%–60% of homeless patients recorded alcohol dependence. These patients frequently do not receive welfare, are disconnected from a social network including families, and are unable to use available social services. They often enter treatment through intervention by church groups, 12-step programs, and after-hospital detoxification. Clinics that work with homeless substance abusers struggle with trying to get basic social support services with adequate provision for meals and a place to live.

■ MINORITIES

Alcohol abuse and drug abuse are major problems in subsets of minority populations (24). SUDs have had a major impact on overall life expectancies in blacks, Hispanics, and Native Americans. Although blacks have comparable rates of heavy drinking compared with whites, blacks have suffered a disproportionate amount of medical, psychological, and social sequelae. Blacks have twice the rate of cirrhosis of the liver and 10 times the rate of esophageal cancer in the 35- to 44-year-old age group. Hypertension is also a greater problem for black patients. Half of black homicide cases are alcohol related. The rates of substance abuse may be skewed somewhat due to statistics that rely heavily on public facilities. Blacks and Hispanics make up 12% and 7%, respectively, of the U.S. population, but they make up 26% and 14%, respectively, of the people with AIDS. Excessive alcohol consumption is also reported among rural and urban Native Americans.

Targeting Treatment

Several researchers have been working in the area of minority substance abuse; however, there has been a paucity of information and data vitally needed in this area. It cannot be assumed that research and program design applicable to middle-class white Americans will be equally applicable to minority communities. There is a recognition of the need for culturally sensitive treatment programs in minority communities. The meaning of the term *culturally sensitive* is open to research and discussion. There are some culturally specific etiologic and treatment-related problems. Unemployment, racism, poor self-esteem, corruption of cultural values, and economic exploitation are prevailing problems in urban black communities and may contribute to the high rates of psychoactive substance abuse. Blacks are more readily diagnosed with alcoholism than are whites and are often misdiagnosed psychiatrically. Black teenagers report less alcohol abuse than white teenagers. However, blacks have comparable rates of abuse in their 20s and 30s. Although the biopsychosocial approach is equally valid with minorities, social factors such as poor education, unemployment, low job skills, racism, and substance-abusing peer role models become important etiological factors and should be addressed in any culturally sensitive program. Recognition and cooperation of indigenous cultural institutions such as churches are needed. Blacks have had less access to treatment in the past; cutbacks in funding of social agencies may further block access to treatment. Family treatment approaches are especially valuable in the Hispanic community. The importance of respect for cultural diversity is essential in drug treatment programs.

Cultural Patterns

Parties in which alcohol is consumed to excess and disinhibition is sanctioned (the concept of the *drinking party*) are a prevalent aspect of Native American culture. In Hispanic culture, a macho notion in which manhood is equated with the ability to hold one's liquor may be prevalent. If a man is able to provide for his family, alcoholism may be well tolerated. Alcohol is often seen as a celebration of life and integrally related to holidays and festivals. Exposure of alcoholism often brings shame to the family and the community.

Treatment in minority communities generally must focus more on the extended family. Treatment programs and AA meetings must have some flexibility and respond to cultural norms. The heterogeneity within the minority communities must also be recognized. For example, rural southern American blacks may have different cultural norms compared with West Indian blacks. In addition, minority women may have different roles and special treatment issues that are not prevalent in the majority population. In family therapy with Hispanic groups (e.g., families), attention to issues related to respect and machismo lead to good results. There are unmet needs for Native Americans with substance abuse problems, and we must address why and take measures to correct this (25).

In summary, treatment personnel are faced with combining good basic alcohol and drug abuse treatment with cultural sensitivity. In reality, alcohol and drugs are going to remain a major problem within minority communities until we adequately address basic social ills.

■ REFERENCES

1. Warner LA, Kessler RC, Hughes M, et al: Prevalence and correlates of drug use and dependence in the United States. Arch Gen Psychiatry 52:219–228, 1995

2. Ashley MJ, Olin JS, LeRiche WH, et al: Morbidity in alcoholics: evidence for accelerated development of physical disease in women. Arch Intern Med 137:883–887, 1977

3. Eronen M: Mental disorders and homicidal behavior in female subjects. Am J Psychiatry 152:1216–1218, 1995

4. Kessler RC, Sonnega A, Bromet E, et al: Post-traumatic stress disorder in the national comorbidity survey. Arch Gen Psychiatry 52:1048–1060, 1995

5. Blume S: Addictive disorders in women, in Clinical Textbook of Addictive Disorders, 2nd Edition. Edited by Frances RJ, Miller SI. New York, Guilford Press, 1998

6. Urbano-Marquez A, Ramon E, Fernandez-Sola J, et al: The greater risk of alcoholic cardiomyopathy and myopathy in women compared with men. JAMA 274:149–154, 1995

7. Longnecker MP, Berlin JA, Orza MJ, et al: A meta-analysis of alcohol consumption in relation to breast cancer. JAMA 260:652–656, 1988

8. Gavaler JS, Rizzo A, Rossaro L, et al: Sexuality of alcoholic women with menstrual cycle function: effects of duration of alcohol abstinence. Alcohol Clin Exp Res 17:778–781, 1995

9. Brown HL, Britton KA, Mahaffey D, et al: Methadone maintenance in pregnancy: a reappraisal. Am J Obstet Gynecol 179:459–463, 1998

10. Volpe JJ: Effect of cocaine use on the fetus. N Engl J Med 327:399–407, 1992

11. Institute of Medicine: Fetal alcohol syndrome: research base for diagnostic criteria, epidemiology, prevention, and treatment. Washington, DC, National Academy Press, 1995

12. American Academy of Child and Adolescent Psychiatry: Practice parameters for the assessment and treatment of children

and adolescents with substance use disorders. J Am Acad Child Adolesc Psychiatry 36:140S–156S, 1997

13. O'Malley PM, Johnston LD, Bachman JG: Adolescent substance use: epidemiology and implications for public policy. Pediatr Clin North Am 42:241–260, 1995

14. Bachman JG, Wallace JM Jr, O'Malley PM: Racial/ethnic differences in smoking, drinking, and illicit drug use among American high school seniors, 1976–89. Am J Public Health 81:372–377, 1991

15. DeWit DJ, Adlaf EM, Offord DR, et al: Age at first alcohol use: a risk factor for the development of alcohol disorders. Am J Psychiatry 157:745–750, 2000

16. Blood L, Cornwall A: Pretreatment variables that predict completion of an adolescent substance abuse treatment program. J Nerv Ment Dis 182:14–19, 1994

17. Biderman J, Wilen T, Mick E, et al: Is ADHD a risk factor for psychoactive substance use disorders? findings from a four-year prospective study. J Am Acad Child Adolesc Psychiatry 36:21–29, 1997

18. Kaminer Y: Adolescent Substance Abuse: A Comprehensive Guide to Theory and Practice. New York, Plenum, 1994

19. Botvin GJ, Baker E, Dusenbury L, et al: Long-term follow-up results of a randomized drug abuse prevention trial in a white middle-class population. JAMA 273:1106–1112, 1995

20. Humphreys K, Moos RH: Reduced substance-abuse-related health care costs among voluntary participants in Alcoholics Anonymous. Psychiatr Serv 47:709–713, 1996

21. Saunders PA, Copeland JRM, Dewey ME, et al: Heavy drinking as a risk factor for depression and dementia in elderly men. Br J Psychiatry 159:213–216, 1991

22. Abrams RC, Alexopoulos GS: Substance abuse in the elderly: over-the-counter and illegal drugs. Hosp Comm Psychiatry 39:822–823, 1988

23. Koegel P, Burnam A: Alcoholism among homeless adults in the inner city of Los Angeles. Arch Gen Psychiatry 45:1011–1018, 1988

24. Franklin J: Minority populations, in Clinical Textbook of Addictive Disorders, 2nd Edition. Edited by Frances RJ, Miller SI. New York, Guilford Press, 1998

25. Novins DK, Beals J, Sack WH, et al: Unmet needs for substance abuse and mental health services among northern plains American Indian adolescents. Psychiatr Serv 51:1045–1047, 2000

INDEX

*Page numbers printed in **boldface** type refer to tables or figures.*